PANDEMIC

We're not so different

We may have different views but the difference is not wide
And policies of hate just serve to divide
So let us talk and we may see
That we're not so different, you and me.
Please don't judge by colour, creed or gender
Instead let's love each other
And lend a helping hand to friend or foe
And anger, hurt and misery will simply up and go
Let us pass on to others once in a while
A simple courtesy and a willing smile.

PRG 14.6.2020

PANDEMIC
2nd Edition: Conspiracies and Cover-ups!

Paul R Goddard
MD, BSc, MBBS, DMRD, FRCR, FBIR, FHEA

with contributions from
Nabil Jarad
Lois Tutton
Angus Dalgleish
and
photography by

Mark Goddard
Lois Goddard
Chris Holder
Jerome Tilleul
Ian Crighton
Peter Dougill
Damien Cheung
Brian Joannidi

Laura Hildebrandt

© **Paul R Goddard 2020 / 2021**

The right of Paul R Goddard to be identified as the author and artist of this work has been asserted by him in accordance with the Copyright, Designs and Patents Act 1988.

All rights reserved. No part of this publication may be reproduced, stored in a retrieval system, or transmitted in any form or by any means, electronic, mechanical, photocopying, recording or otherwise, without prior permission from the copyright owner.

While the advice and information in this book is believed to be true and accurate at the time of going to press, neither the author, the editor, nor the publisher can accept legal responsibility for any errors of omissions that may be made. The publisher makes no warranty, express or implied, with respect to the material contained herein. Case histories and names have been altered to preserve confidentiality.

First published in the UK June 2020.
Revised for the 2nd edition September 2021

A catalogue record for this book is available from the British Library

ISBN: 978-1-85-457105-2

PANDEMIC: 2nd Edition: Conspiracies and Cover-ups
Published by:
Clinical Press Ltd.
Redland Green Farm, Redland, Bristol, BS6 7HF

****

About the Author

Paul R Goddard is emeritus Professor of Radiology at the University of the West of England and a retired consultant and head of training from the Bristol Royal Infirmary. His interests include painting, composing, playing in a jazz band and lecturing on the history of the horrible plagues that beset human beings.

Professor Goddard wrote his first book in 1987 entitled "Diagnostic Imaging of the Chest" and published by Churchill Livingstone. He has published many books and research papers since then and the first edition of this book was published in June 2020.

He won the Couch Award, the Kodak Scholarship and the Twining Medal from the Royal College of Radiologists and the Barclay Prize and Honorary Fellowship from the British Institute of Radiology.

Contents

	Page No.
About the author	4
Acknowledgements	6
Foreword by **Professor Angus Dalgleish**	7
Professor of Oncology, St George's Hospital, London	
Preface	8

Chapter

1. Introduction, The World's Worst Pandemics ... 9
   Correlations between plagues and war.
2. Smallpox ... 20
3. Malaria ... 26
4. The Bubonic Plague ... 30
5. Tuberculosis ... 40
6. Influenza ... 53
7. Syphilis, Lyme Disease, Leprosy ... 61
8. Diarrhoea and Dysentery: Cholera, Typhoid, Typhus and more... 71
9. The AIDS epidemic and hepatitis ... 82
10. It's an infection but it's not what you think! ... 87
11. Coronavirus: The Origin of the COVID-19 Virus ... 91
12. Coronavirus: The COVID-19 Pandemic ... 106
13. Coronavirus: The Responses to the COVID-19 Pandemic ... 117
14. Coronavirus: The effects of lockdowns ... 123
15. Coronavirus: Treatments for COVID-19 ... 148
16. Coronavirus: Vaccines against COVID-19 ... 156
17. Antibiotics and Vaccination lead to complacency ... 163
18. A Far Future Plague and Conclusions ... 171
    Index ... 176

Acknowledgements

At the start of the COVID-19 outbreak I posted a few comments on Facebook and a somewhat comical song on Youtube. These were received with some amusement and interest and the response of my friends has encouraged me to finish writing the book on pandemics and plagues that I had started a few years ago. In particular I would like to thank the support given by my wife, Lois and my two sons, Jeremy and Mark. Their comments, ideas, photographs and general encouragement has been outstanding.

Thank you to Jessie Smithson for the rainbow on the back cover and on page 139 and to Ian Daley who, on his own, kept the Redland Minimarket food store open seven days a week throughout the lockdown.

Nabil Jarad, Lois Tutton and Angus Dalgleish have discussed COVID-19 with me from the outset and contributed to several chapters in the 2nd edition.
Thank you.

In addition, and in random order, I acknowledge the support on Facebook and elsewhere provided by:

Francis Smith, Simon Best, Chris Holder, Jeremy Mann, John and Anne Gane, Jerome Tilleul, Ian Crighton, Peter Dougill, Arvind Chaturvedi, Damien Cheung, Moses T Jones, Nick Blanch, John Lyall, Stephen, Alison and Sam Goddard, Sarah Nkansah Michaels, Kristy Thomson, Paul Savoie, Chris Grieve, Liz Varley, Lydia Cuadrat, Sarah Carr, Keith Carr, Liz Beckman, Nick Thomson, Dave Robert Page, Sonja Maas, Chris Daws, Graham Daws, Sanjiv Nandi, Barry Nicholson, Maha Elias, Deenagh Miller, the Crowthers, Peter Fifield, Jim Farrell, Scarlett Stone, Lynda Lee, Rod Symmons, Dewinder Bhachu, Robert Burch, Joy Storey, Nicola Smith, Hazel Storey, John Graham, Benjamin Brown, Laura Drury, James Harris, Christian Walsh, Hal Crafer, Julian Warren, Emma Birth, Fiona Cranmore, Ian Benton, Nate Goody, Al Cosnett, George Grimble, Orinn Checkley Freediver, Andrew Gibbs, James Harris, Glen Scott, Vasilli Papastravou, Julian Lea-Jones, Al Cosnett, Stuart Green, Emma Yelding, John Graham, Pat Turton, Bridget Barker, Ali Bayman, Jonathan Pitts-Crick, David Adams, Laura Varley, Dave Collas, Sanjay Prabhu, Graham Smith, Andrew Smith, Sandra Zealand, Peter Bruce, Jane Williams, Mick Daws, Pam Bayman, Niall Monaghan, John Christopher Brooks, Abbie Connors Atkinson, Dee Jeffries, David Brown, Brain and Judy Joannidi and many more.

Not all of them are relatives or in my pay!

Foreword to the First Edition

This book is incredibly timely coming as it does at the end of the COVID-19 lockdown in the UK and elsewhere. It reviews the history of pandemics in a very balanced way going into detail on the top 10 of all time.

As well as being full of useful facts placed in context with regards to history, each disease is graced with a list of famous sufferers. The author enlivens each chapter with personal experiences and anecdotes. Indeed his experience working in Africa on his elective and a working lifetime in the NHS make him well placed to put many of these disease in context including malaria, leprosy, tuberculosis and HIV.

Such a book could easily come across as merely a history of plagues, but not this one. The author has the surprising ability to grab the reader's interest with his own cartoons and scattered throughout are pictures of famous or in some cases not so well known sufferers of the diseases described or the doctors who have made such a difference in overcoming these maladies.

The narrative glides into a diary of the current COVID-19 pandemic and examines all the relevant issues including how did it ever occur in a world which was meant to have leadership from the WHO to protect us from these dramatic black swan events? Just when you thought that would be a great ending to this book there follows a series of dramatic photographs to bring home the effect of this on our society.

But the revelations do not end there, he proposes that the other serious pandemic of dementia may have more to do with a common bacterial infection affecting our gums than the prion hypothesis, and moreover how to avoid it.

A very welcome focus on how vaccines and medications have revolutionised the management of the great scourges such as smallpox and the plague is followed by a chapter which I suspected might be missing from this book. This is computer viruses and the fact that they also represent a very real potential nightmare scenario for us all.

This volume is simultaneously informative and amusing in a style that only a superb polymath like Paul Goddard can do. I can't wait for his next book as he can turn his hand to anything including writing great songs and music and fascinating novels which again I cannot put down until I have finished them!

Angus Dalgleish MD, FRCP, FMedSci
Professor of Oncology, St George's Hospital

Preface

Preface for PANDEMIC: 2nd Edition: Conspiracies and Cover-ups!

The first edition of PANDEMIC was already half-written before the advent of the coronavirus pandemic which has now killed over four million people worldwide. At the time of writing the section on COVID-19 I noted that the pandemic was still in progress around the world so the story was bound to change. Even still I felt that a blow by blow account of life in the first lockdown in living memory was a worthwhile endeavour and since the book had to be reprinted due to demand it seems that other people also felt it was of value.

Now, after 130,000 deaths in the UK (which is a further 69,000 deaths after the first wave) we appear to have the virus under control in the UK by dint of a mass vaccination programme. For this we must thank the people working in the NHS, a veritable army of volunteers and the scientists who made the vaccines.

Unfortunately there is rarely a straightforward plot in real life. As they say "truth is stranger than fiction". The people who make vaccines are both the heroes and the villains. Evidence is emerging that the COVID-19 virus is the product of experimentation on a bat coronavirus. I will present evidence that the virus was created in one of the three virology laboratories in Wuhan, China. Astonishingly the research was funded by the National Institutes of Health of the USA, led by Dr Fauci, who passed the money to Peter Daszak of EcoHealth Alliance, thence to the Chinese virologist, Shi Zhengli. Thus they enabled the techniques of Gain of Function studies to be applied to bat coronaviruses in the Chinese laboratories in collaborative projects that have been extensively written up. The exact experiment and the exact coronavirus which created the SARS2 COVID-19 virus, out of over two hundred viruses that were being played with, has not been discovered although a very similar virus to COVID-19 was immediately identified. What is apparent is that the only intermediate animal was not a poor pangolin but a laboratory humanized mouse. Moreover it is almost impossible to infect bats with the COVID-19 and no examples of wild bats infected with it have been found.

So what has the response to this information been? Almost universal denial by virologists who all failed to admit their conflict of interests. The chapters on COVID-19 have been considerably expanded and now include sections on the origin of the virus, the actual pandemic and the variants, the mixed response around the world including lockdowns, self-isolation and quarantine, repurposed drugs, vaccines, the outcome and the burden of COVID-19 affecting health, wealth and well-being. I also ask what should be done to stop future mistakes of this nature. Some of the other chapters have been slightly adapted. My tasteless cartoons have been increased in number. Sorry about that!

Paul R Goddard   July 2021

Chapter 1

As I write this book the world is *still* in the grip of a pandemic: the SARS2 COVID-19 coronavirus. But, perhaps contrary to expectations, this book was not written because of the virus. I was already writing it based on the Long Fox Lecture I had delivered to the Bristol Medico Chirurgical Society, on November 8th, 2017 and I have, of course, updated it with reference to the present pandemic. Moreover, like many other people, I was already warning people about future pandemics including a specific mention of novel coronaviruses. I was very pleased to have been asked to give the 2017 Long Fox lecture. I considered this to be a singular honour. So I shall start by explaining three good reasons why *Pandemics: Plagues, Pestilence and War* was appropriate as title and subtitle for the first edition of this book. The subtitle has been changed to *Conspiracies and Cover-ups!* and the reasons will become apparent as you read the newer sections.

Firstly: I believe that **Dr. Long Fox** would have approved.

Edward Long Fox (1832 – 28 March 1902) was physician to the Bristol Royal Infirmary for some twenty years [1]. I quote now from the inaugural Long Fox lecture, delivered in 1904 by Dr. John Beddoe MD, also formerly physician to the Bristol Royal Infirmary [2].

"A few years after he had begun practice, a serious epidemic of typhus fever broke out in the lower parts of East Bristol. There was no organisation ready to meet and cope with such a calamity…The better educated people in the slums - nurses and Bible readers and the like - stayed in their posts, but the infection was very fatal among them - brains are a disadvantage in true typhus….Edward Fox…created an organisation to meet it…the plague was stayed and doubtless many lives were preserved."

Secondly: I present here in cartoon form, **"President Trump"**. President Trump was elected on November 8th 2016, exactly one year to the day before the presentation of the lecture and was still in office when the first edition of this book was published. He was beaten in the US election of 2020 by Jo Biden. The last trump is described in the Book of Revelation of St. John the Divine.

"They were given power over a fourth of the earth to kill by sword, famine, plague, and by the wild beasts of the earth." [3]

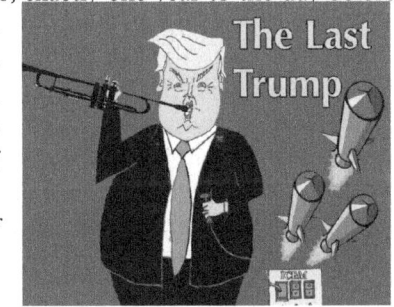

Trump was not responsible for the present pandemic sweeping the world. His trade war with China may or may not have been a contributory factor. See Chapter 11 for a tasteless cartoon of the Chinese premier. My poorly drawn cartoons are in most of the chapters. It's a serious subject so you need a little light relief!

Thirdly: **the hubris of medical scientists and doctors.** On the front cover of New Scientist in 2017 it stated *"The Next Plague: We don't know where it's coming from but we know how to beat it."* [4] That hardly seemed credible when you see the headline in the New Scientist in September 2017. *"Thousands of new lifeforms discovered that redraw the tree of life."* [5] Using the Polymerase Chain Reaction (PCR) twenty new phyla have been discovered revealing the fact that only 5% to 10% of organisms in the soil and in the sea have previously even been named yet alone investigated. *"DNA analysis has unmasked thousands of them and made life's story far more complex"* [5]. The same problem arises with pneumonia.....the organism causing the chest infection is only identified in just over half of the cases and in many people the doctors do not even bother to try to grow the bug that has caused the disease, relying instead on antibiotics and our immune systems to sort out the problem.

The present crisis due to the COVID-19 pandemic has brought to the attention of the public problems with the way that we are responding to epidemics. After the discovery of the germ theory of disease by Pasteur (and others) and, just before the advent of antibiotics, the importance of tracing contacts, isolating and quarantining were well known and carefully observed.

Quarantine as a method of preventing the spread of an infectious disease, goes back to Biblical times.[6] The word comes from the Italian Quarantina, meaning a period of forty days and initially it meant exactly that.[7] People suspected or known to have come into contact with an infectious disease were put in complete isolation for six weeks. This particularly became significant with the Bubonic Plague.

Other diseases that prompted people to isolate themselves or led others to quarantine them included smallpox, leprosy, syphilis, tuberculosis and even streptococcal infections in the form of the dreaded scarlet fever. A reduction in our fear of pandemics started with Jenner's promotion of vaccination (1796) followed by the twentieth century discovery of antibiotics. It became "obvious" that many infections could be treated with either oral or intravenous therapy and if they could not be cured that way they could be prevented by immunisation. We gradually lost our dread of contagion and began to think that infections were nothing to worry about.

We were hopelessly wrong!

The present pandemic at the time of writing, (SARS 2 (COVID-19)), has hammered this home to the public but other recent pandemics should have alerted us. HIV and the AIDS epidemic, the Ebola crisis in Africa, SARS and MERS....these should have warned us.

Plagues and pestilence particularly affect history by wiping out whole armies and even by killing the leaders of countries in conflict. But does it also work the other way round? Do wars, revolution and famine, due to man's inhumanity to man, predispose to pandemics? Are many pandemics fostered by mans' inhumanity?

Another important question is this. To what extent are epidemics and pandemics caused by animal diseases, otherwise called zoonotic infections?

Is this becoming more important and, if so, why?

In this book I will present lists of the worst pandemics in world history and of famous people killed by plagues. Correlation of epidemics with wars and conflicts suggests that the suggestion above is true and that wars and revolutions, man-made famines and disasters, and encroachment on the habitat of animals may indeed lead on to plagues and pandemics. Correlation is not proof of causation and it is not possible to undertake a double blind, randomised crossover trial on a subject such as this. So you will have to look at the evidence and make your own mind up.

Examples of medical staff dying from infectious diseases they are trying to treat are also presented in the book. It is not a new phenomenon.

Thousands of people have died prematurely because the lessons of history have not been heeded. This book is a short, personal history of pandemics, what conditions are likely to cause them and what can be done to prevent or alleviate them. Then, near the end, I give a run-down on the COVID-19 crisis and what I think could be done, even now. And there is one more chapter on a major pandemic you probably do not realise is due to an infection. You may need to take an anxiolytic in order to finish this book. Oh..I forgot, the use of such props has almost become a plague in itself.

205. SMALL POX.

Drink largely of toast and water.

Or, let your whole food be milk and water, mixed with a little white bread.

Or, milk and apples.

Take care to have free, pure and cool air. Therefore open the casement every day; only do not let it chill the patient.

If they strike in, and convulsions follow, drink a pint of cold water immediately. This instantly stops the convulsion, and drives out the pock.— Tried.

"There may be pustules a second time, coming out and ripening like the small pox, but it is barely a cutaneous disorder.

"In violent cases, bleed in the foot; bathe the legs in warm water twice or thrice a-day, before and at the eruption, and apply boiled turnips to the feet. Never keep the head too hot.

"In very low depressed cases wine may be given, and if the pustules lie buried in the skin, a gentle vomit; in many cases a gentle purge of manna, cream of tartar or rhubarb.

"In the Crude Ichorose small pox, a dish of coffee now and then, with a little thick milk in it, has often quieted the vexatious cough.

"After the incrustation is formed, change the sick, but let it be with very dry warm linen.—*Dr. Huxham.*

206. A LONG RUNNING SORE IN THE BACK.

Was entirely cured by eating betony in every thing.

Or, take every morning two or three spoonsful of nettle juice, and apply nettles bruised in a mortar

Treatment of Smallpox
(John Wesley's Primitive Physic 1847)

Definitions of the words Plague and Pandemic

'**The plague**: *a contagious bacterial disease characterized by fever and delirium, typically with the formation of buboes and sometimes infection of the lungs*' ⁽⁸⁾. *Bubonic plague (also pneumonic and septicaemic forms)*

'**Plague:** *Any contagious disease that spreads rapidly and kills many people. Diseases like smallpox wiped out the indigenous people in a succession of plagues.*'

'**Pandemic:** *(of a disease) prevalent over a whole country or the world*'⁽⁸⁾

Factors Affecting Spread of Infections

The World Health Organisation has stated that: '*A number of environmental factors influence the spread of communicable diseases that are prone to cause epidemics.*' ⁽⁹⁾

According to the WHO the most important of these are:
- water supply
- sanitation facilities
- food
- climate.

Many of the largest pandemics have taken the world by surprise and the above stated factors were not particularly the cause. Stephen Morse has described '*Factors in the Emergence of Infectious Diseases*' ⁽¹⁰⁾

'*Emerging infectious diseases are those that have newly appeared in a population*'.... '*ecological, environmental, or demographic factors that place people at increased contact with a previously unfamiliar microbe or its natural host or promote dissemination.*'

I am adding that to create a pandemic you must have:
1. An organism that is sufficiently contagious or spread sufficiently by a vector
2. A large enough reservoir of infection in the original host community
3. Unusual movement of people into an area where the population has no resistance to the disease or weakening of the population by previous disease, starvation, war or deprivation.

I will present the evidence for this in the rest of this book and that Samuel von Pufendorf was right when he wrote: "*More inhumanity has been done by man himself than any other of nature's causes.*" ⁽¹¹⁾ This, of course, has been paraphrased as "*Man's inhumanity to man*", first documented in a Robert Burns poem called *Man was made to mourn: A Dirge* in 1784.⁽¹²⁾

Plagues in History

How is it possible to know about plagues that pre-date written history?

There are three main ways of discovering more about ancient pandemics.

- Language: word of mouth leading to very early writings.
- Pictures: carvings/paintings
- Bones and fossils, x-rays and unwrapping of mummies, DNA sampling of bones and teeth etc.

The study of ancient nucleic acid (aDNA) has accelerated due to the use of the Polymerase chain reaction (PCR). PCR is a technique that takes a single copy or a few copies of a piece of DNA and amplifies it into millions of copies.

The worlds worst pandemics

A list is presented here of the world's worst pandemics of an individual infection. Some of the figures are conjectures or *"best guess"* as we are often dealing with ancient history. Even today it is difficult to get precise figures of mortality caused by infections such as malaria.

They are presented in reverse order in the best tradition of TV reality shows and beauty contests!

The World's Ten Worst Pandemics in Reverse order

-10-
Hepatitis

By 2013 Hepatitis C had risen above HIV, Tuberculosis and Malaria in the annual world ranking of causes of death. Many of the patients with Hepatitis C were infected by medical treatment, vaccinations, blood transfusion etcetera.

Fortunately treatment is now available: ledipasvir–sofosbuvir. Unfortunately the cost of an eight-week course is £26,000 and a 12-week course is £39,000 (plus VAT). An additional drug that may be needed is called ribavirin. Some people may need a 24-week course, costing £78,000. The UK's National Health Service (NHS) is rationing these drugs such that only the sickest patients get them. [13,14].

-9-
Syphilis

"In 1495 an epidemic of a new and terrible disease broke out among the soldiers of Charles VIII of France when he invaded Naples in the first of the Italian Wars, and its subsequent impact on the peoples of Europe was devastating – this was syphilis, or grande verole, the "great pox." [15]

-8-
Epidemic Typhus

In Russia, during the civil war between the White and Red Armies (1917-1922), typhus killed 3 million people, mainly civilians. During World War II, many German POWs after the loss at Stalingrad died of typhus. [16]

-7-
Cholera

Cholera Deaths in India between 1817 and 1860, in the first three pandemics of the nineteenth century, are estimated to have exceeded 15 million people. Another 23 million died between 1865 and 1917, during the next three pandemics. Cholera deaths in the Russian Empire during a similar time period exceeded 2 million. [17]

-6-
HIV/AIDS

Since 1980, the beginning of the epidemic, more than 70 million people have been infected with the HIV virus and about 35 million people have died of HIV [18]

-5-
Spanish Flu

Starting near the end of the First World War in 1918 and extending through to 1920, between 50 to 100 million people died from the so-called Spanish Flu (H1N1 influenza virus) [19]

-4-
Tuberculosis

Tuberculosis (TB) is still one of the top ten causes of death worldwide.

In 2016, 10.4 million people fell ill with TB and 1.8 million died from the disease (including 0.4 million among people with HIV). Over 95% of TB deaths occur in low and middle income countries (WHO). Globally, the TB mortality rate fell by 37% between 2000 and 2016. [20] In the middle of the 19th century during the Industrial Revolution up to one third of Londoners died from tuberculosis.

-3-
Bubonic Plague (The Plague)

The three major pandemics of the Plague (Bubonic and Pneumonic):
- Justinian Plague: 541 AD, killed 50-60% of the European population.
- The Black Death: 1347-1351...killed 60% of Europe's population (some say more)
- "Third Pandemic" : This began in China in 1855 and killed twelve million people in Asia. [21]

The subject of the Plague will be addressed later in this book.

-2-
Malaria.

About 3.2 billion people – almost half of the world's population – are at risk of malaria. In 2013, there were about 198 million malaria cases (with an uncertainty range of 124 million to 283 million).

It is estimated that there are 584,000 malaria deaths per annum (with an uncertainty range of 367,000 to 755, 000)(WHO). [22]

And now for Number One
The most deadly pandemic!

####### 1 #######
Smallpox

Smallpox killed more than three hundred million people in the 20th century alone. That's 300,000,000 ! Two million died as recently as 1967 (WHO). [16]

Smallpox killed a large proportion of the native Americans, perhaps 80 to 90% and the latest research suggests that it almost entirely wiped out the sophisticated civilisation living in the Amazon rain forest.

The Antonine Plague of AD 165 killed five million or more…..The list goes on and on. Smallpox was eradicated in 1979 but note well: it is still kept alive in two laboratories, one each in the United States and Russia, from whence it could be weaponised.

Also Ran... (The runners up)

That's the top ten individual diseases causing pandemics but using other ways of assessing problems will give a different answer. For example, grouping together all the gastro-intestinal diseases causing catastrophic diarrhoea (eg. typhoid, paratyphoid, cholera, typhus, shigella, amoebiasis, norovirus, enterobacter, E.coli …..) would make diarrhoea number one *. Or look at the certified reported causes of death and one might assume that pneumonia was first on the list of pandemics even though the organisms causing death are endemic in the population and are rarely identified individually on the certification and in the developed world the pneumonia usually occurs when the individual is near death from some other condition such as heart failure or metastatic disease.

There are many diseases that can or might cause pandemics but arguably not resulting in death frequently enough to rise into the top ten. The following is an incomplete list of such diseases in no particular order:

- COVID-19 (Sars-2) : over 4 million killed worldwide since 2019
- Yellow Fever
- Diphtheria
- Measles
- Typhoid
- Polio
- Leprosy
- Lyme disease
- Coronaviruses
- Scarlet Fever
- Haemorrhagic Viruses: Filoviridae (Filovirus) Ebola and Marburg
- The mystery disease in chapter 10!

* Note: Although an 'Also Ran' bowel motions are often referred to as number two, not number one!

Ten correlations between Plagues and War

Plagues, pestilence, and pandemics in general, particularly accompany war.

I have listed below ten good examples of pandemics occurring because of war but it is a historic fact that World War 1 (WW1) was the first war in which more people died on the battlefield than from disease off the battlefield and even then the flu epidemic took over at the end of the war and killed more people after the war than died in the war. Starvation and famine is a factor in this story. People affected by siege, starvation, lack of sleep, grief and horror have weakened immune responses and succumb to infection. Big population movements, such as occur during wars due to movement of armies and displacement of people as refugees, spread disease. Destruction of the infrastructure destroys the water supplies and sewage facilities. Read on:

1. The biggest single population devastation from smallpox occurred during the conquest of the Americas by the Spanish.
2. The Hundred Years' War was a series of conflicts waged from 1337 to 1453. Black Death broke out in 1347.
3. Spanish flu broke out towards the end of WW1 when the soldiers were exhausted and many thousands of Chinese workers had been employed to remove the bodies and clear up the battlefields.
4. A new genetic history of HIV shows how the Aids pandemic probably originated in about the 1920s in Kinshasa in the Democratic Republic of Congo. Leopold II's administration of the Congo Free State became one of the greatest international scandals of the early-20th century. It had led to the death of perhaps 20% of the population (10 -15 million people) by 1908.
5. The Justinian plague broke out during wars to retake the Roman Empire
6. The Third pandemic broke out in China between the two Opium Wars (1855)
7. Tuberculosis was the principal cause of death in 1650 (civil war in Britain) but probably reached a peak in the middle of the Industrial Revolution.
8. Syphilis first appeared in Europe after the conquest of the Americas
9. Cholera and Typhus are closely associated with wars, revolutions and disasters.
10. The plague of Athens (probably Typhoid, evidenced from DNA in the teeth) occurred during the Peloponnesian War 430BC.

Malaria seems indifferent to hostilities, killing with or without wars. It did, however, tend to keep invading armies away from Rome. The local people, including the incumbent pope, had some immunity to the endemic malaria but invaders did not.

In the next few chapters....

This small book does not purport to be a textbook of infectious diseases.

The intention of the book is to permit the reader to discern patterns in the way that pandemics occur and how the plagues alter history and history alters plagues. In the next few chapters we give a little more detail about the infections that cause pandemics and provide a list of the famous people who died from those diseases. Look out for the occasional names of doctors who died from the contagious diseases they were trying to treat.

References

1. Edward Long Fox, https://en.wikipedia.org/wiki/Edward_Long_Fox_(physician)
2. The Long Fox lecture, John Beddoe. The Bristol Medico Chirurgical Journal 22, 303-320, 1904
3. Book of Revelation of St John the Divine 6 verses 7-8, The Holy Bible, New American Standard Bible (NASB)
4. New Scientist 25th February 2017
5. New Scientist 10th September 2017
6. (https://en.wikipedia.org/wiki/Quarantine)
7. (https://www.dictionary.com/e/quarantine-vs-isolation/)
8. Pages dictionary
9. http://www.who.int/environmental_health_emergencies\/d/isease_outbreaks/communicable_diseases/en
10. Stephen Morse "Factors in the Emergence of Infectious Diseases Emerging" Infectious Diseases1995;1 (1) 7-15 https://wwwnc.cdc.gov/eid/article/1/1/95-0102_article
11. Samuel von Pufendorf The Whole Duty of Man According to the Law of Nature 1673
12. Robert Burns, Man was made to mourn: A Dirge 1784
13. New data shows relentless rise in hepatitis deaths. http://www.who.int/hepatitis/news-events/WorldHepatitisSummit2015-PressRelease.pdf
14. NHS 'abandoning' thousands by rationing hepatitis C drugs https://www.theguardian.com/society/2016/jul/28/nhs-abandoning-thousands-by-rationing-hepatitis-c-drugs
15. Syphilis - its early history and treatment until penicillin, and the debate on its origins Frith, John, Journal of Military and Veterans Health.Volume 20 Issue 4 (Dec 2012)
16. Typhus- https://en.wikipedia.org/wiki/Epidemic_typhus
17. Cholera: https://en.wikipedia.org/wiki/Cholera_outbreaks_and_pandemics
18. HIV/AIDS, WHO http://www.who.int/gho/hiv/en/
19. https://en.wikipedia.org/wiki/1918_flu_pandemic
20. WHO Global Tuberculosis Report 2017   http://www.who.int/tb/publications/factsheet_global.pdf
21. The Justinian Plague, Paul R Goddard, Proceedings , Bristol Medico-Historical Society, Volume 5, pp 107-112 ISBN 9780952704751
22. WHO Fact sheet on the World Malaria Report 2014 December 2014.http://www.who.int/malaria/media/world_malaria_report_2014/en/
23. Worst Killer Plagues in history https://www.oddee.com/item_90608.aspx

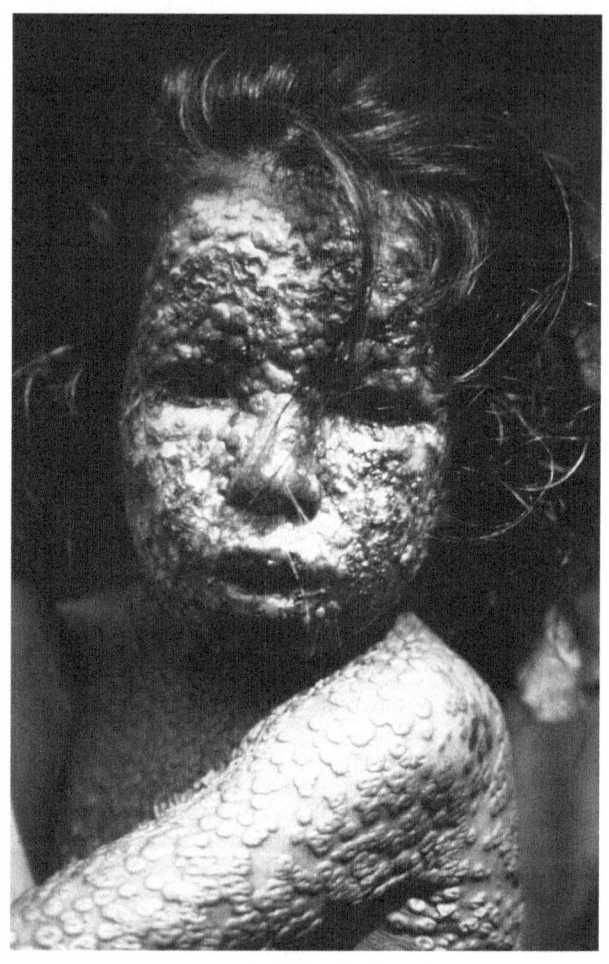

This young girl in Bangladesh was infected with smallpox in 1973. Freedom from smallpox was declared in Bangladesh in December, 1977 when a WHO International Commission officially certified that smallpox had been eradicated from that country.

Patients with ordinary-type smallpox usually had bumps filled with a thick and opaque fluid, often with a depression or dimple in the center. This is a major distinguishing characteristic of the disease.

(Content Providers(s): CDC/James Hicks/Wikipedia [1]

Chapter 2
Smallpox

As discussed in the last chapter it is probable that smallpox in a series of pandemics or endemic in the population has killed more people than any other single disease with the possible exception of malaria.

Smallpox is an acute viral disease caused by the variola virus. It occurred in two forms, variola minor and variola major. Originally known, in England, as "the red plague" or just as "the pox" it was re-named smallpox after the advent of syphilis in the fifteenth century.

It is considered likely that smallpox affected the ancient Egyptians judging from smallpox-like lesions on the skin of some mummies.[2] Indeed the mummified head of Ramases V shows evidence of the disease.[3,4] The disease probably spread via trading routes to Asia and is described in early Chinese and Indian texts.

The Antonine plague of 166 AD, also known as the plague of Galen, was mentioned in Chapter 1. This was a pandemic brought back to the Roman Empire by troops returning from besieging Seleucia of Mesopotamia. The plague killed up to a third of the population of the Roman Empire.

As trade opened up around the world, smallpox went with it.[5]

The Center for Disease Control and Prevention (CDC) have provided an interesting list of smallpox "historical highlights".[5]

- 6th Century – Increased trade with China and Korea introduces smallpox into Japan.
- 7th Century – Arab expansion spreads smallpox into northern Africa, Spain, and Portugal.
- 11th Century – Crusades further spread smallpox in Europe.
- 15th Century – Portuguese occupation introduces smallpox into part of western Africa.
- 16th Century – European colonization and the African slave trade import smallpox into the Caribbean and Central and South America.
- 17th Century – European colonization imports smallpox into North America.
- 18th Century – Exploration by Great Britain introduces smallpox into Australia.

It was well known that variola minor had a much reduced mortality rate compared with variola major, probably less than 1%. Inoculation (variolation) using the minor variety was used as a preventive measure in China as early as the tenth century[6]. It was introduced to the UK in 1717 but Drs Robert and

Daniel Sutton reported in 1760 that in 30,000 inoculation cases there were 1200 fatalities.

Near the end of the 18th Century Edward Jenner made one of the most important discoveries in medical science. Jenner noted that milkmaids in Gloucestershire, England, having contracted the mild condition known as cowpox from infected nipples of cows, believed that they were subsequently immune to smallpox.

The beauty and healthy nature of milkmaids was legendary, probably because they did not suffer the ravages of smallpox. In the late 1790s Jenner subcutaneously inoculated patients with the milder cowpox virus successfully in twenty-three trial cases.

Parliament in 1802 and 1807 voted Jenner £30,000 to improve and spread his method.[7,8] This was one of the most significant State interventions in the history of medical science and Jenner's technique has undoubtedly saved countless millions of lives.

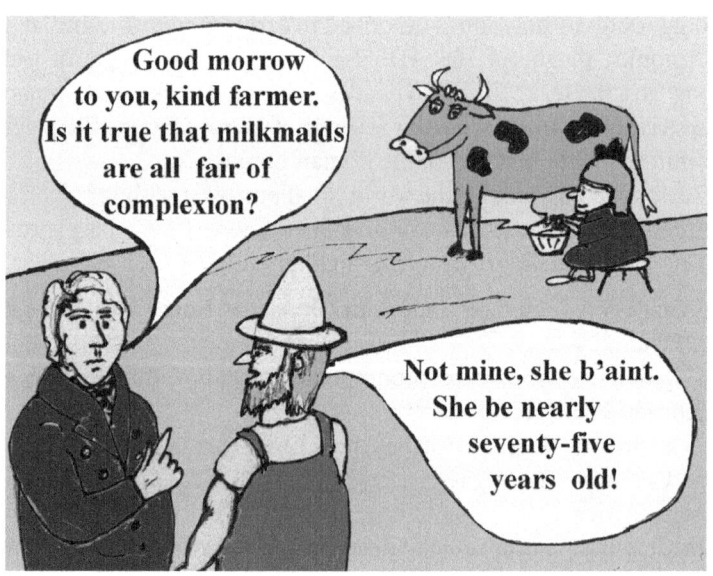

Jenner enquires about the beauty of milkmaids

Smallpox Weaponised?

In 1971 an outbreak (10 cases, 3 fatal) of smallpox involved a ship from Araisk which had sailed near a Soviet weapons facility near Vozrozhdeniiye Island in the Aral Sea. This may have been an escape of the virus from a laboratory or a deliberate release of weaponised smallpox. Systematic vaccination of all people in the vicinity prevented a major epidemic in the Soviet Union.[9]

The Last Cases

The last case of "wild" smallpox was contracted in Somalia in 1977. However, in tragic circumstances the last person to die from the disease did so in Birmingham, England. The patient's name was Janet Parker (1938–1978), a British medical photographer. She was working in a small office above a Biosafety Level 4 laboratory growing the strain of smallpox which killed her. Five hundred people were quarantined as contacts but the only other person to catch the disease was her mother, who survived. The head of the laboratory committed suicide and Janet's father died of a cardiac arrest when visiting her in hospital. Apallingly a similar outbreak had occurred originating from the same laboratory in 1966.[10]

On December 9, 1979, the Global Commission for the Certification of Smallpox Eradication signed their names to the statement that *"smallpox has been eradicated from the world."*

Very many famous people must have died from smallpox. Here are just a few. [11]

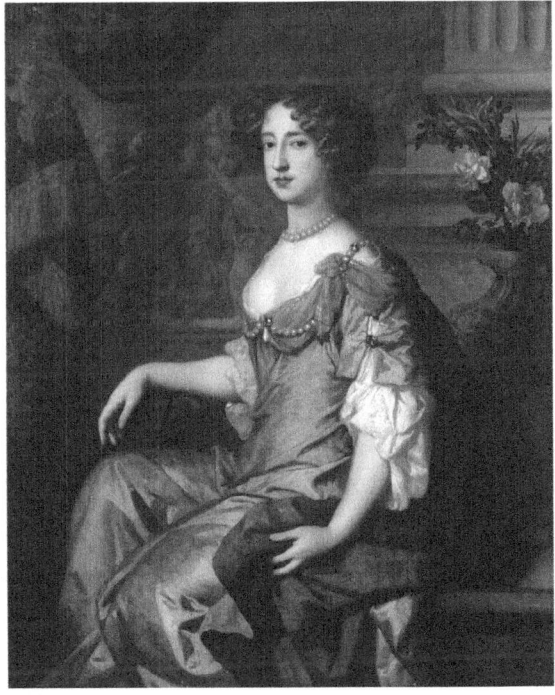

Mary II of England
(1662-1694)

Mary ruled England, Wales, Scotland and Ireland jointly with her husband William III. They displaced her father, James II of England, VII of Scotland, at the "Glorious Revolution" of 1688.

In late 1694, however, she contracted smallpox. She sent away anyone who had not previously had the disease, to prevent the spread of infection and died in Kensington Palace. (Wikipedia [12])

Louis XV of France (1710 – 1774), known as Louis the Beloved. Reigned until his death from smallpox. He was the first Bourbon ruler whose heart was not, as tradition demanded, cut out and placed in a special coffer. The body was not embalmed for fear of contamination; instead, alcohol was poured into the coffin. The remains were also soaked in quicklime.

In a late-night ceremony attended by only one courtier, the body was taken to the Saint Denis Basilica. (Wikipedia [13])

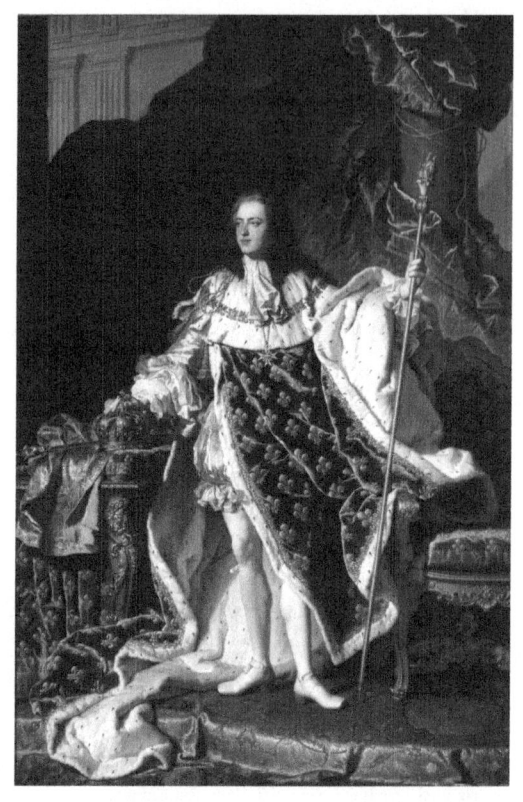

Peter II of Russia

Born 1715 Peter II Alexeyevich reigned as emperor of Russia for under three years. In December 1729 he fell ill, dying on 30th January 1730 from smallpox, the very day he had planned to marry Ekaterina Dolgorukova [14]

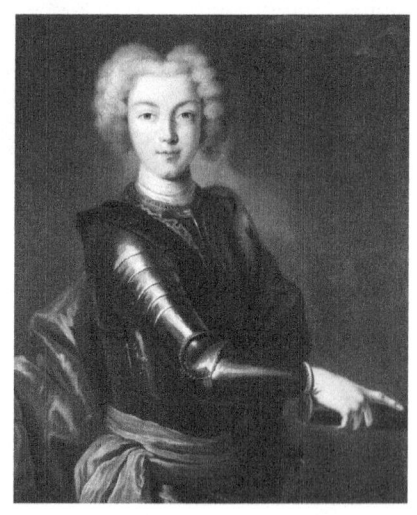

Geeta Bali started her film career as a child actress, at the age of 12, with the film The Cobbler. She made her debut as a heroine in Badnaami (1946) becoming a star in the 1950s. She starred in more than 70 films in a 10 year career.

She died on 21 January 1965, having contracted smallpox while shooting a Punjabi film, Rano, based on a novel Eik Chadar Maili Si by Rajinder Singh Bedi. [15]

Movie stills from Naya Ghar cropped on Geeta Bali: D. D. Kashyap (Director-Producer) [15]

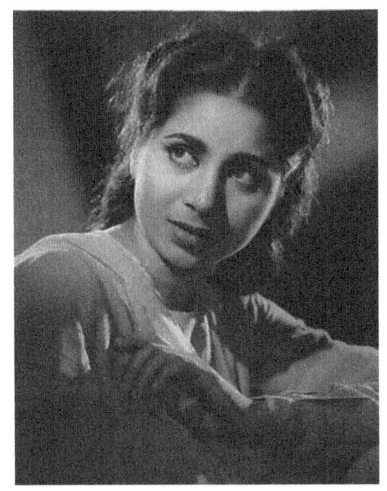

References

1. Girl with smallpox CDC/James Hicks/Wikipedia Reference: https://en.wikipedia.org/wiki/Smallpox)
2. https://www.cdc.gov/smallpox/history/history.html).
3. https://www.ncbi.nlm.nih.gov/pmc/articles/PMC1200696/
4. Lyons AS, Petrucelli RJ., II . New York: Abradale Press, Harry N Abrams Inc; 1987. Medicine—An Illustrated History
5. https://www.cdc.gov/smallpox/history/history.html
6. https://en.wikipedia.org/wiki/Smallpox
7. The history of medicine, money and politics, P Goddard 2008, Clinical Press.
8. The Age of Napoleon pp392-393
9. https://en.wikipedia.org/wiki/1971_Aral_smallpox_incident)
10. https://en.wikipedia.org/wiki/1978_smallpox_outbreak_in_the_United_Kingdom
11. https://www.ranker.com/list/famous-people-who-died-of-smallpox/reference
12. https://en.wikipedia.org/wiki/Mary_II_of_England#Reign
13. https://en.wikipedia.org/wiki/Louis_XV_of_France#Death
14. https://en.wikipedia.org/wiki/Peter_II_of_Russia
15. https://en.wikipedia.org/wiki/Geeta_Bali

Chapter 3
Malaria

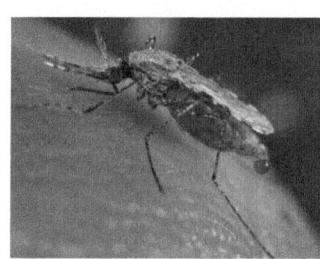

An Anopheles stephensi mosquito obtaining a blood meal from a human host through its pointed proboscis. Note the droplet of blood being expelled from the abdomen after having engorged itself on its host's blood:
CDC/ Dr. William Collins, Jim Gathany [1]

In 1974 I spent three months in Zaria, Nigeria, working with another medical student at Wusasa Missionary Hospital. We acted as locum doctors looking after outpatients, performing surgery and attending the patients on the wards. In particular we had many children dying from infectious diseases including measles and malaria. Every day an infant or child would die, usually from measles bronchopeumonia, for which nothing could be done, or from malarial meningitis, which was also nigh impossible to treat even with anti-malarial drugs. As I write this I know that very sadly the frontline staff in the NHS are dealing with daily mortality due to the COVID-19 coronavirus pandemic and my experiences in Africa were the nearest that I got to that kind of heart-breaking scenario. My thoughts are with the NHS staff.

As stated in Chapter 1 of this book almost half of the world's population are at risk of malaria. Half a million people die from the disease each year. The disease is caused by parasitic protozoans (single cell organisms) of the Plasmodium type. Five species of Plasmodium can infect and be spread by and to humans. P. falciparum is the most dangerous form and causes most of the fatalities. P. vivax, P. ovale and P. malariae generally cause a milder form of malaria.[2,3,4]

The species P. knowlesi only occasionally infects human beings. The disease is transmitted from person to person by mosquitoes acting as a vector. The usual vector is a female Anopheles mosquito.

Malaria is now mainly found in tropical countries and is therefore considered to be a tropical disease. This was not always the case and the mosquitoes that carry malaria are found all over the world. Malaria has been eradicated from much of the developed world but the last indigenous case in England was in the 1950s, USA 1950s and Holland 1961. The World Health Organization declared Italy free of malaria on November 17th 1970 and the whole of Europe in 1975. Australia was declared free of indigenous malaria as late as 1981.

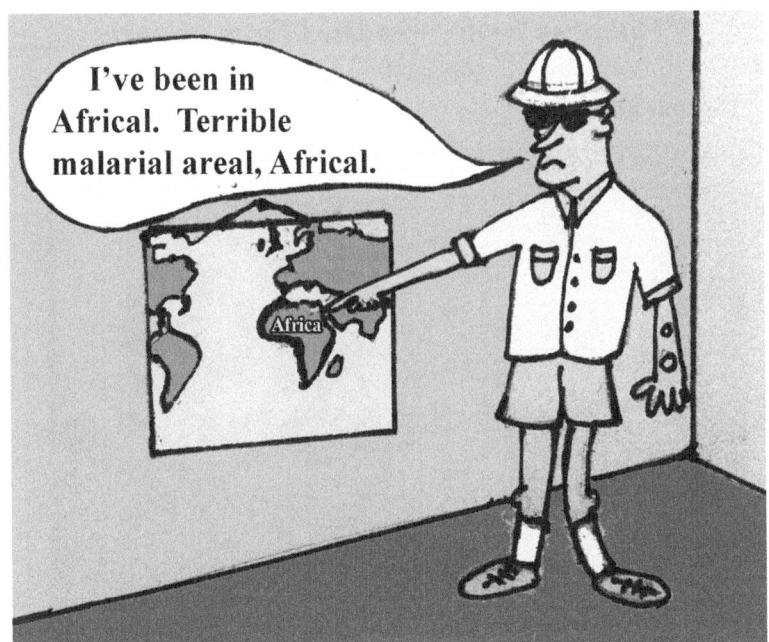

Above: Bristol explorer returns home having noted the high incidence of malaria in Africa*

*Note: Bristolians are famous for adding the letter L to the ends of words that end in a vowel. The name Bristol is said to derive from Brycgstow (plus, of course, the L). The above sentence was spoken to a hospital doctor in Bristol in 1990.

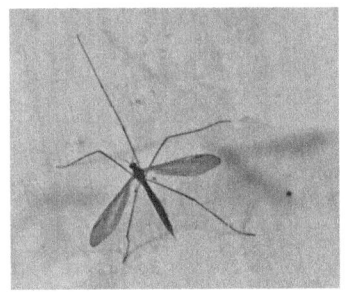

Right: Anopheles mosquito in Bristol (June 2020)

Most malaria cases and deaths occur in sub-Saharan Africa. However South-East Asia, Eastern Mediterranean, Western Pacific and Central and South America are also at risk.

Artemesinin

In 1972 Tu Youyou was heading a project in China to find a new anti-malarial treatment. Drug companies in the West had screened one quarter of a million compounds without success but Tu decided to study Chinese herbal medicines. One was effective: sweet wormwood (*Artemisia annua*) used for 'intermittent fevers'. The extract is now called Artemesinin and, in combination with other anti-malarials, has saved countless lives. Tu Youyou shared the Nobel Prize for Medicine or Physiology in 2015.

Famous People Who Died From Malaria[5]
Kings/Popes etc.

- Genghis Khan

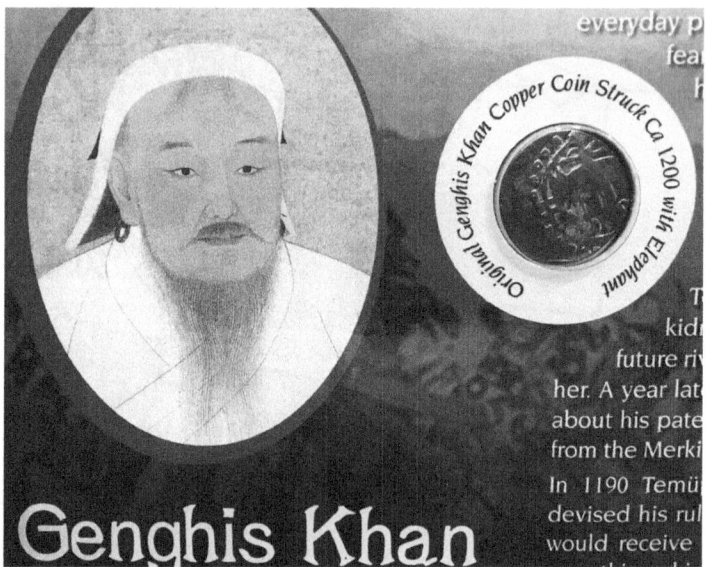

Original Genghis Khan coin
Purchased from Coincraft, London in presentation packet

Genghis Khan suffered from a type of malaria in the spring of 1227 while nursing battle injuries.

After several months of sickness, the Great Khan died at the age of around sixty years old. Scientists from the Russian Academy of Scientists believe that he has 16 million descendants living today.

- Oliver Cromwell 1599-1658

Cromwell was an English general who led the armies of the English parliament in the civil wars against Charles I. He became Lord Protector of the Commonwealth.

He died aged fifty-nine from malaria contracted whilst fighting in Ireland.

Oliver Cromwell shilling

Some other famous leaders who died from malaria.
- Colonel Prince Henry of Battenberg Died at 38 (1858-1896)
- Pope Urban VII Died at 69 (1521-1590)
- Giovanni de' Medici the Younger Died at 18 (1544-1562)
- Henry VI Holy Roman Emperor from 1191 until his death. Died at 32 (1165-1197)
- Otto III Holy Roman Emperor (June/July 980 – 23 January 1002)
- Conrad IV King Of Germany and Sicily Died at 26 (1228-1254)
- Louis III was titular King of Naples 1417–26 Died at 31
- Possibly Alexander the Great

Famous people who died from Malaria.
- Amerigo Vespucci Died at 58 (1454-1512)
- Mary Livingstone Died at 41 (1821-1862)
- David Livingstone Died at 60 (1813-1873)

Marsh Wives

The Romans famously drained the swamps to reduce the "miasma" they believed caused disease and in doing so markedly reduced the mosquito population and malaria.

The fate of Marsh Wives was well known in England from the sixteenth to the eighteenth centuries. The population of the Fens and the coastal regions of Essex and Kent was considerable and the farmers wealthy. Their wives, often from London or further away, were not as lucky as the farmers. The locally born inhabitants had some resistance to Marsh Fever but the wives did not and succumbed after a short time of wedded bliss. The farmer would then travel to the big city and find another happy bride. Some farmers got through fifteen wives![6] It was not until the 1830s that the mortality levels began to fall.[7]

References

1. Mosquito photograph from CDC/ Dr. William Collins, Jim Gathany https://phil.cdc.gov/details.aspx?pid=5814
2. Caraballo H (2014). "Emergency department management of mosquito-borne illness: Malaria, dengue, and west nile virus". Emergency Medicine Practice. 16 (5). Archived from the original on 2016-08-01.
3. "Malaria Fact sheet N°94". WHO. March 2014. Archived from the original on 3 September 2014. Retrieved 28 August 2014.
4. https://en.wikipedia.org/wiki/Malaria
5. http://www.ranker.com/list/famous-people-who-died-of-malaria/reference
6. The mosquito: A human history of our deadliest predator. Timothy C Winegard
7. Contours of Death and Disease in Early Modern England, Dobson and Smith 2003

Chapter 4
The Bubonic Plague

Researchers have extracted Plague DNA from the teeth of Bronze age people who lived **5000 years ago**[1]. Yersinia pestis became transmissible by fleas c.**1000BC**.

Three pandemics have been identified and will be discussed here

The Justinian Plague 540 AD
The Black Death 1346 AD
The Third pandemic 1850 AD

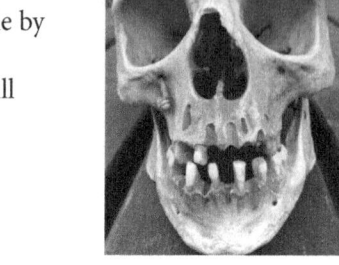

Right: Justinian Gold Solidus

Above: Ancient skull

The First Pandemic

The first Pandemic is known as the Justinian Plague because it occurred in the reign of the Eastern Roman Emperor of that name who ruled the empire from **527-565AD**. He was a very able administrator who set up the Justinian legal code which was adopted by much of Europe and was only superseded by Napoleonic law one thousand and three hundred years later.

Justinian had excellent generals working for him and an efficient army. They had defeated the Persian Empire, retaken north Africa, Spain and part of Italy. In doing so he killed a *'myriad of myriads of people**.'[2,3]

The Roman Empire was very much in business again and we in Europe might still be under the rule of the Empire if a series of tragedies had not struck. An enormous volcanic eruption at the site of the present day Krakatoa was followed by sunless summers and widespread crop failures. Tree ring analysis from this era shows ten years with no growth.

Historians Flavius Cassiodorus, Procopius (Byzantine Historian) and Michael the Syrian all recorded in **536AD** that the sun had lost its power.

John of Ephesis wrote "There was a sign from the Sun, the likes of which had never been seen or reported before. The Sun became dark, and its darkness lasted for about 18 months. Each day, it showed for about four hours and still this light was only a feeble shadow. Everyone declared that the Sun would never recover its full light again.

---

*Note: myriad: An unspecified but exceedingly large number. A multitude.

In China the *'stars were lost from view for three months.'* The famine was followed by a terrible outbreak of Bubonic Plague. This spread from the East into Europe. In **542 AD** plague broke out in the capital of the Empire, Constantinople. The plague was reported to have begun in central Asia, spread into Egypt, and then made its way through Europe reaching Britain by **547AD**

This is the first recorded pandemic that can with any certainty be ascribed to Bubonic Plague

Symptoms started with hallucinations, fever and fatigue with some people suffering from a sore throat and diarrhoea. These symptoms soon led on to the characteristic sign of Bubonic Plague: swellings or buboes in the groin and armpits. These suppurated or became gangrenous. Death occurred in the vast majority affected.

Procopius (Byzantine Historian) recorded that at its peak the plague was killing 10,000 people per day in Constantinople.[2]

As the world's first known pandemic spread throughout the empire (and beyond) the military campaigns of Justinian faltered and failed. At home Justinian had to suppress revolts against increased taxes.

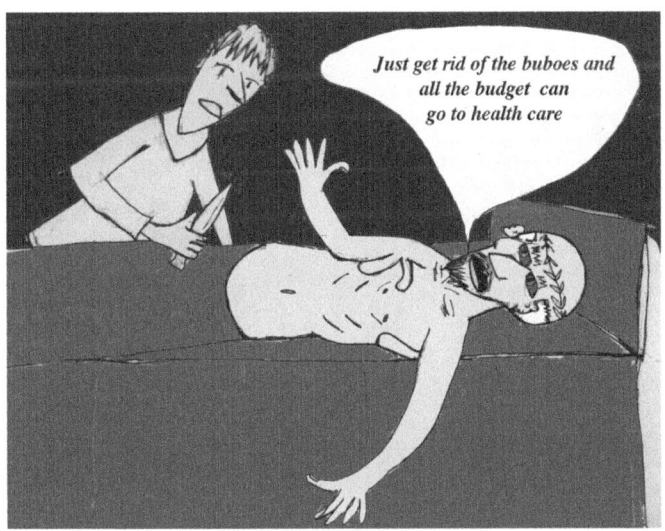

Justinian is treated by the physician/surgeon Sampson

The plague and the failed military adventures led to financial ruin of the empire and even the emperor Justinian caught the plague!

Justinian was treated successfully by Sampson (later called St Sampson), a physician from Rome. In gratitude the emperor built him a large hospital: The Hospice of St Sampson.

Some historians such as Josiah C. Russell have suggested a total European population loss of 50 to 60 percent between **541 AD** and **700 AD**

The Justinian plague and the subsequent waves of the plague which affected each generation, were seen as evidence of God's wrath against sinful leaders and wicked people. In Europe the Roman Catholic Church gained ascendancy over rational argument for 1000 years, controlling all aspects of life including medicine. In the East it can be argued that the power vacuum permitted the rise of Islam.

The Second Pandemic: The Black Death

This pandemic is said to have started in Mongolia. The disease made its way to Europe in **1346**. In one famous incident, the Tatars, a group of Mongolian Turks, were battling Italians from Genoa in the Middle East when the Tatars were suddenly stuck down by the plague. Reportedly, they began catapulting dead bodies over the Genoans' walls toward their enemy, who fled back to Italy with the disease.

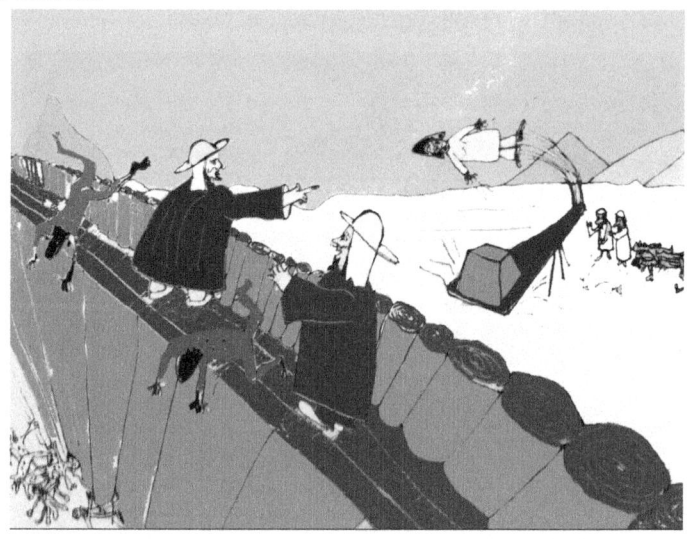

First defender (pointing): If they throw any more dead bodies at us I'm going home
Second defender: Genoa?
First defender: Never seen her before in my life

The incurable plague known as the 'Black Death' swept across Europe killing at least a third of the population. Conservative estimates say it killed seventy-five million of the World's 450 million population but it was very probably many more. It is likely that the Black Death was a variant of Bubonic/Pneumonic plague but it has some unusual features.

The Black Death arrived in Britain on the **25th June 1348** through Weymouth. This is documented in the Grey Friars Chronicle

"In this year 1348 in Melcombe, in the county of Dorset, a little before the feast of St. John the Baptist, two ships, one of them from Bristol came alongside. One of the sailors had brought with him from Gascony the seeds of the terrible pestilence and through him the men of that town of Melcombe were the first in England to be infected."

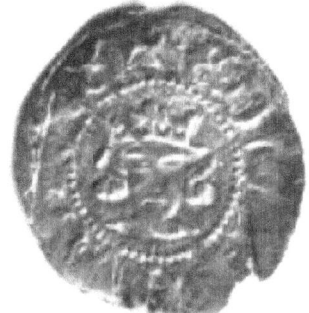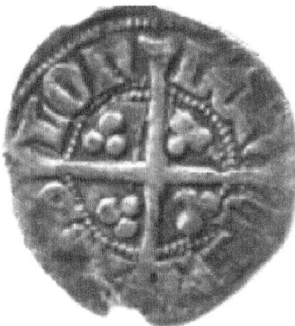

Edward III silver penny (x2 diameter)

Edward III ordered that movement of people from Weymouth should be restricted. It was too late. The Death spread to Bristol and then to London and the rest of Britain. Geoffrey le Baker, a contemporary cleric of Oxford wrote: '*And at first it carried off almost all the inhabitants of the seaports in Dorset, and then those living inland and from there it raged so dreadfully through Devon and Somerset as far as Bristol and then men of Gloucester refused those of Bristol entrance to their*

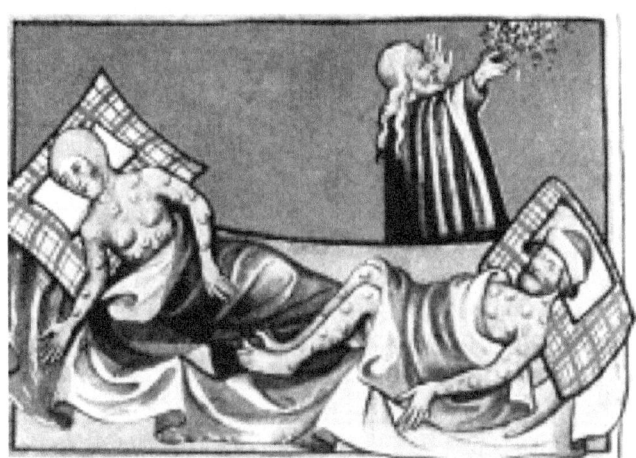

Illustration of the Black Death from the Toggenburg Bible (1411)

county, everyone thinking that the breath of those who lived amongst people who died of the plague was infectious. But at last it attacked Gloucester, yea and Oxford and London, and finally the whole of England so violently that scarce one in ten of either sex was left alive.'

According to an article in the Bristol Medico-Chirurgical Journal[4] of 1894: 'When the plague came there was little power of resistance. Few of those who were seized with it lived as long as three days; many died after one or even half a day's sickness.... The immediate effect of this calamity was a huge immigration of men from country to take up trades, and these gave rise to a distinct wage-earning class with interests and objects apart from their employers. The sudden removal of about half of the population threw great wealth and great possibilities into the hands of the survivors.'

There was a particularly bad outbreak in Bristol in **1564-65** 'a very hot plague' killing two and a half thousand people. The Plague returned periodically until the late 17th century. Famously the plague is remembered in nursery rhymes:

Ring a ring o' roses
A pocket full of posies
Atishoo! Atishoo!
We all fall down

This probably dates to the Great Plague of London 1665

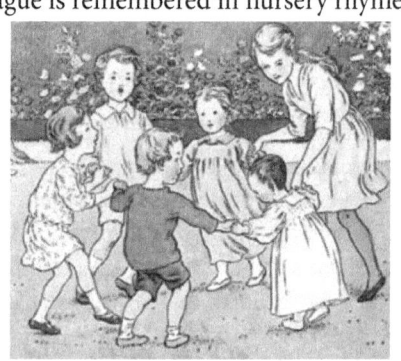

"*Ring a ring o' roses*": the rosy colored rash, appearing on the affected person, as an early symptom of Plague.

"*A pocket full of posies*" : the medicines and herbs people used to carry in their pockets-hoping to keep off the plague

"*Atishoo! Atishoo! We all fall down*": the sneezes of the plague victim before he or she falls down dead.

The sneezes remind us that the plague was not just manifesting as swellings or buboes but also through the highly contagious pneumonic form which killed the victim so quickly and spread like wild fire, not needing the rats which undoubtedly spread the slower, bubonic version.

In a recent report in New Scientist by Anthony King[5] the coronavirus NL63 is mentioned and its ancient leap from bats to man, estimated to have occurred sometime in the 13th to 15th century. Virologist Ralph Baric is quoted as saying '*When it did, the result was probably a pandemic.*' Like SARS-CoV-2 the NL63 virus latches on to the ACE2 receptor and was probably deadly. Baric asks us to search for a pandemic in that era. Perhaps the Black Death is that very pandemic. That the two were spread together would explain a lot. Bacterial and viral co-infection is increasingly recognised as an underlying aetiology in community and hospital acquired pneumonia [6] and is reckoned to have had a part to play in the "Spanish" flu of 1918. The then novel coronavirus NL63, plus Bubonic Plague would have been an extra deadly combination.

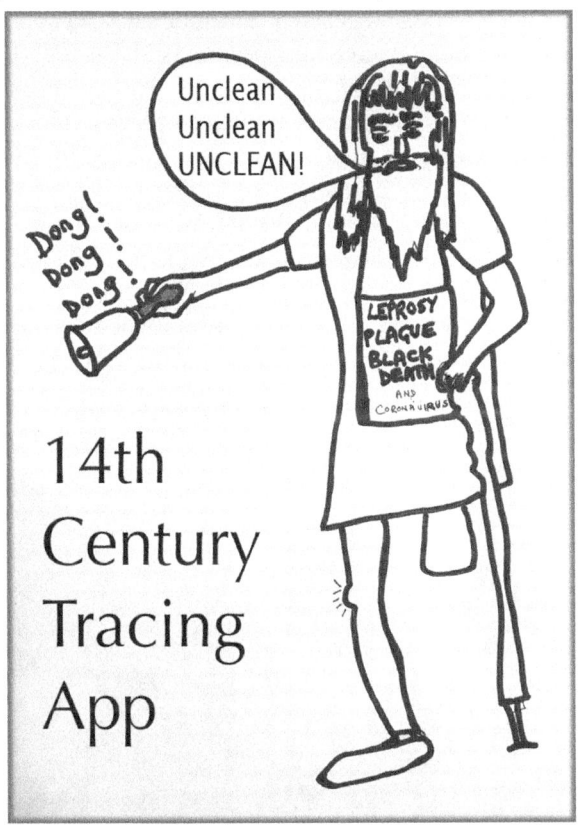

The Plague of **1603** coincided with the accession of James I to the throne of England. The plague began in the parish of Stepney at the time of Queen Elizabeth's death in March and by the date of the coronation of James, July 18th, the deaths had reached 1000 a week. *"The victims came mostly from the crowded lanes of the sinfully polluted suburbs"* wrote James Bamford, minister of St Olave's. He found that the infection was most rife among *"such as do not greatly regard clean and sweet keeping and are pestered together in alleys and houses"*. All those who could flee from the city did so, including almost all the doctors.

James I, a believer in the divine rights of kings but a Presbyterian, was persuaded to continue the practice of 'touching' to cure the King's Evil on the grounds that it would not be a popular act if he stopped what had become a form of 'Royal Health Service'. He presumably did not try 'touching' to cure the plague!

In **1603** one physician who honourably stayed at his post in Warwick Lane was Dr. Thomas Lodge. Lodge was better remembered as a poet having written Rosalynde, the source of William Shakespeare's *As You Like It*. In 1603 Lodge published *A Treatise of the Plague*.[7]

Towards the end of 1603 King James granted a licence to reopen the Curtain and Boar's Head theatres as soon as the plague decreased to thirty deaths per week in London.

The plague of **1625** coincided with the accession of Charles I. Dr Thomas Lodge died when fighting the plague in 1625 and the same plague killed another of Shakespeare's collaborators; John Fletcher (1579-1625).

The Great Plague of London (**1665**) was only stopped by the Great Fire of London of **1666**, having wreaked havoc throughout the country, not just London.

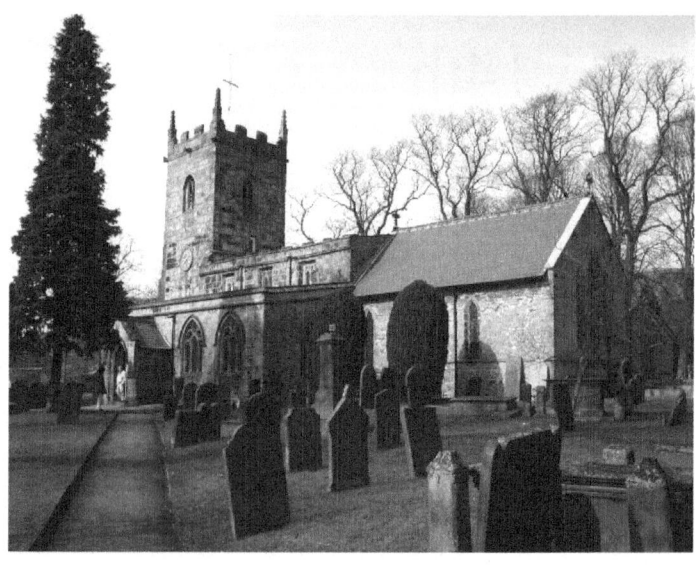

The Church at Eyam

The whole villlage of Eyam in Derbyshire went into self-imposed voluntary quarantine rather than spread the disease. The church has a record of 273 individuals who died from the disease but the villagers' actions stopped the plague from spreading into neighbouring areas.[8]

The Third Pandemic

The 3rd pandemic started in China in 1855 and killed 12 million people in China and India alone. Outbreaks appeared in ports around the world for the next fifty years. The 2nd Opium War, where Britain and France fought China, forcing the Chinese to take our opium in trade, raged between 1856 and 1860.

World War 1 Plague in Bristol 1916

The port of Bristol was threatened by plague from visiting ships in 1901, 1902 and 1909 but the rats were not permitted to reach the shore. In 1916, during the first world war, the disease mysteriously appeared in the centre of Bristol in a rag warehouse.

Lieut-Col. D.S. Davies, (Medical Officer of Health, Bristol) ordered that the contents of the warehouse should be destroyed by fire. The rats were fed to prevent them from migrating and the staff were inoculated against the plague. The bales of rags were disinfected and taken in closed vans to a city destructor. The work took ten days, sixteen tons of disinfectant were used and two tons of lime. Rat catching was carried out for six months in the surrounding area.

9000 rats were caught but no more plague carriers.

WW2

During world war 2 the Imperial Japanese Army Air Service on two known occasions bombed China with infected fleas. These caused epidemics of the Bubonic Plague.

Personal Experience.

I have no direct experience of the Bubonic Plague except receiving immunisation against it. In 1994 I travelled to the Ukraine to head up a medical mission providing health care for the 43rd Rocket Army in the Ukraine as they broke up the nuclear weapons.

In preparation for the trip I received numerous immunisations including one against the plague.

'It's not very effective,' said the doctor as he injected my leg with a syringe full of turbid material. *'But it's the best we've got.'*

The leg ached for several days but I did not catch the plague. Maybe it worked!

Famous People Who Died from the Bubonic Plague

This has mostly been taken from alchemipedia.blogspot.com [9]
Famous People who have died from Bubonic Plague (Yersinia pestis) infection:
- 251 - Hostilian (Gaius Valens Hostilianus Messius Quintus) (Roman Emperor 251 AD)
- 664 - Saint Cedd (Missionary Bishop, Northumbria)
- 775 - Constantinos Copronymos - Emperor, died 14 September.
- 1270 - Louis IX of France.
- 1347- Sir John Montgomery (John de Montgomery) ex Governor of Calais
- 1348 - Andrea Pisano (Architect & Sculptor, Florence) possibly Black Death. [10]
- 1348 - Joan Plantagenet (daughter of King Edward III)
- 1348 - Ambrogio Lorenzetti (Painter, Siena)
- 1348 - Piettro Lorenzetti (Painter, Siena)
- 1349 - Jeuan Gethin (Welsh Poet)
- 1349 - John de Ufford (sometimes John de Offord or John Offord; Chancellor, Archbishop of Canterbury)
- 1349 - Ralph de Swantone (Priory Infirmarer, Norwich Cathedral)
- 1349 - Sir John Pulteney (Master Draper, 4x Mayor of London)
- 1349 - Thomas Bradwardine (Archbishop of Canterbury)
- 1361 - Lord Reginald Cobham (one of Edward III's leading commanders)
- 1361 - One of the native Irish kings succumbed.
- 1363 - Matteo Villani (brother of Giovanni Villani)
- 1394 - Anne of Bohemia (Wife of King Richard II)
- 1476 - Regiomontanus (mathematical & astronomical prodigy)
- 1505 - Jacob Obrecht (great Dutch Composer)
- 1538 - Family of Nostradamus' (Astrologer) - wife & 2 children.
- 1558 - Joan, elder sister of William Shakespeare.
- 1543 - Hans Holbein the Younger (famous miniature painter)
- 1576 Titian (Painter)
- 1579 - Father of Caravaggio
- 1638 - Adriaen Brouwer (Flemish painter, ? died of the plague).
- 1698 - Catholic Archibishop Pjetër Bogdani (Kosovo)
- 1713 - Prince Paul I. Esterházy

William Shakespeare family members who died of bubonic plague:

- Sisters Joan, Margaret (just babies) & Anne (aged 7).
- Brother Edmund (aged 27).
- Son, Hamnet, who died aged eleven years old

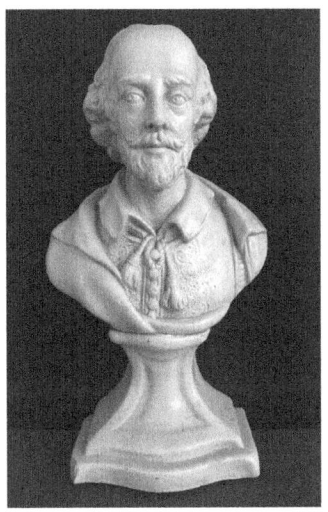

William Shakespeare 1564-1616
The Bard himself died from a fever very suddenly having had a merry meeting with Drayton and Ben Johnson and "it seems drank too hard" [10]

Famous Medical Staff who died from the Plague
- 1625 Dr Thomas Lodge
- 1645 John Paulitious (Edinburgh's first official plague doctor)
- 2009 Professor Malcolm Casadaban (Molecular geneticist and plague researcher).

References

1. Early Divergent Strains of Yersinia pestis in Eurasia 5,000 Years Ago Cell Volume 163, Issue 3, p571–582, 22 October 2015 Rasmussen et al
2. Procopius History of the Wars 545
3. Edward Gibbon The History of the Decline and Fall of the Roman Empire 1776-1788
4. Bristol Medico-Chirurgical Journal 1894 Vol 12 p271
5. An Uncommon Cold, Anthony King New Scientist pp32-35 2.5.2020
6. Pneumonia with bacterial and viral coinfection, Cawcutt, Kelly, Kalil, Andre C. Current Opinion in Critical Care: October 2017 - Volume
7. The History of Medicine, Money and Politics, Paul R Goddard, Clinical Press Ltd. p39 2008
8. https://Wikipedia.org/wiki/Eyam
9. http://alchemipedia.blogspot.com/2009/09/bubonic-plague-famous-deaths.html
10. Quote from John Ward vicar of Stratford in https://Wikipedia.org/wiki/William_Shakespeare

Chapter 5
Tuberculosis

Earliest Evidence of Tuberculosis (TB)

Tuberculosis has been a scourge of humankind from the dawning of civilisation.In 2008, evidence for tuberculosis infection was discovered in human remains from the Neolithic era dating from 9,000 years ago.

Tuberculosis has claimed its victims throughout much of known human history and reached epidemic proportions in Europe and North America during the 18th and 19th centuries, earning the nickname, *"Captain among these Men of Death."*[1]

Thomas M. Daniel in The history of tuberculosis tells us that it is likely that a version of Mycobacterium tuberculosis was present in East Africa three million years ago. The modern strains evolved from a common ancestor around twenty thousand years ago and there are now six major lineages which probably diverged between 250 and 1000 years ago. [1]

Whilst there is no mention directly of tuberculosis (TB) in Egyptian papyrii there is *"abundant archeological evidence"* that it was prevalent in Egypt 5,500 years ago. In addition the typical deformities of spinal TB (Pott's Disease) are found in mummies and are depicted in early Egyptian art. [2] (see below)

Tuberculosis is mentioned in the Old Testament books of the Bible, Leviticus and Deuteronomy, using, in the Authorised Version, the old term for TB, consumption. The ague and fever probably refer to malaria.

"I will even appoint over you terror, consumption and the burning ague." [3]
"The Lord shall smite thee with a consumption and with a fever." [4]

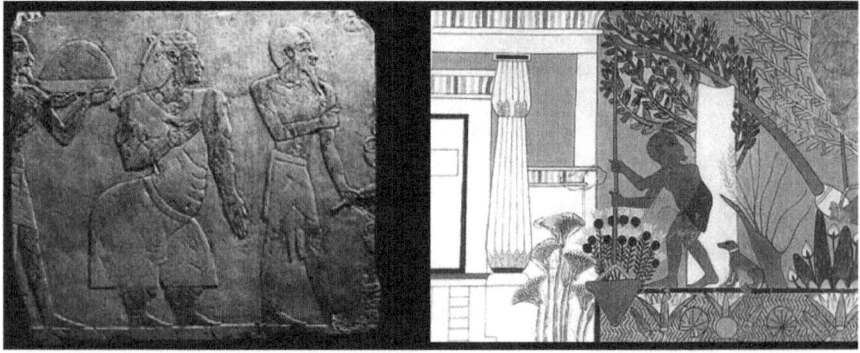

Typical deformities of the spine in ancient Egyptian art
(from Wikipedia)

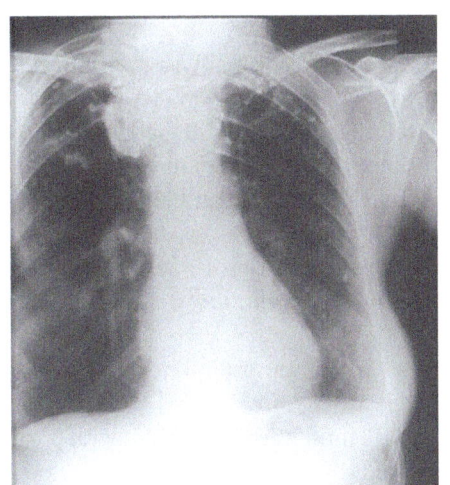
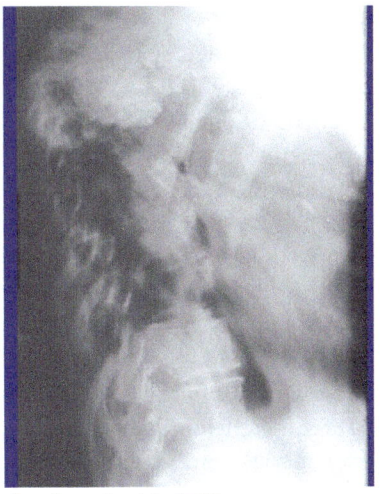

*An example of Pott's Disease in a female patient in 1991
PA and lateral chest radiographs show apical calcification from TB
and deformity of the upper thoracic spine*

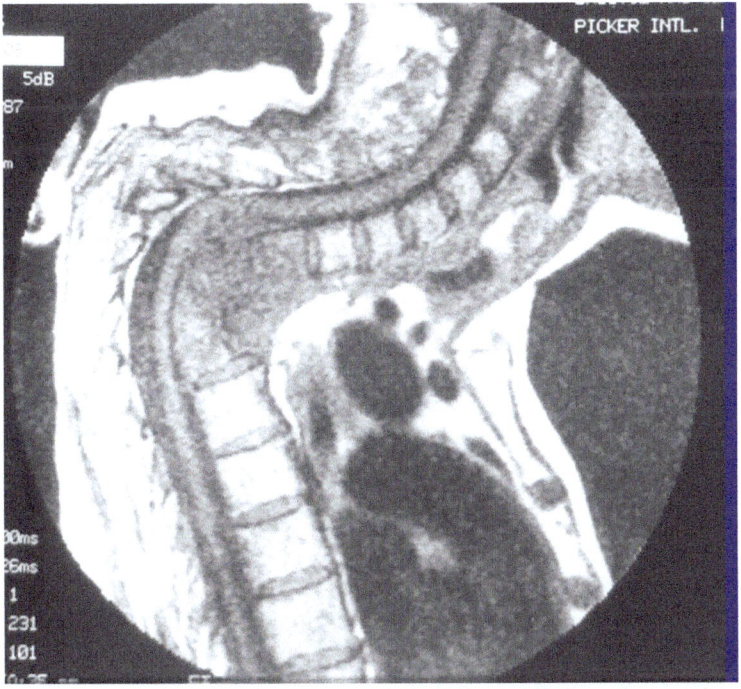

Sagittal T1-weighted MRI of the spine in the same patient shows uncannily similar appearances of bony deformity to those shown in the Egyptian art and compression of the spinal cord by an associated soft tissue mass [5]

Tuberculosis has several names related to its different manifestations. In general in the past it was known as consumption because of the way it consumed the patient. London physician Benjamin Marten suggested in 1790 that it was due to wonderfully minute living creatures[1]. Throughout the next century people made more and more observations to the same effect. Rather than being a romantic disease of people with artistic temperament it was in fact a very nasty infection.

*"In **1838** Chopin was turned away from Palma in Mallorca where he had gone to recuperate from phthisis, (pulmonary TB) on the grounds that it was contagious. He died in Paris in 1849, at the age of 39"* [1]

In **1855** David Livingstone had noted that TB was almost unknown in sub-Saharan Africa until the Europeans arrived.

1865: a French military physician called Villemin injected a rabbit with purulent material from a pleural cavity and showed that tubercles formed in the poor rabbit.

1867: William Budd, Bristol physician, wrote a letter to the Lancet suggesting that tuberculosis *"is disseminated through society by specific germs … cast off by persons … suffering from the disease"*…… He based his view on the epidemiology of tuberculosis.

Portrait of Dr William Budd from an original lithograph published by A.B. Black, 1862, in the Royal Society of Medicine

As well as suggesting that TB was contagious he also described the spread of typhoid and cholera by contaminated water.

Budd's suggestions regarding the germ-based contagious nature of tuberculosis shocked the British medical establishment [6]

Finally Robert Koch convinced the medical world that TB was indeed an infection. Koch, a German physician and scientist, presented his discovery of *Mycobacterium tuberculosis*, the bacterium that causes tuberculosis (TB), on the evening of March 24, **1882**.

He began by reminding the audience of terrifying statistics:
"If the importance of a disease for mankind is measured by the number of fatalities it causes, then tuberculosis must be considered much more important than those most feared infectious diseases, plague, cholera and the like.

One in seven of all human beings dies from tuberculosis. If one only considers the productive middle-age groups, tuberculosis carries away one-third, and often more." [1]

Koch showed that the organism was present in every case of the disease, it could be isolated from a host and grown in culture, samples from the culture caused the same disease when inoculated into a susceptible animal and the organism could be isolated from that animal and identified as being the same as that in the original host. These stages of identification and proof became known as Koch's postulates and have been very important in establishing cause and effect in infectious diseases.

Koch also established the causative agents of cholera and anthrax and received the Nobel prize in Physiology or Medicine in **1905**. [7]

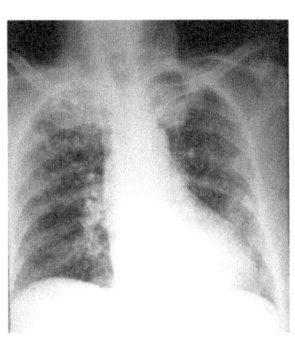
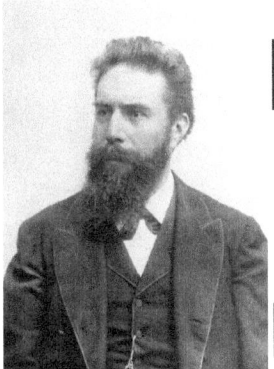
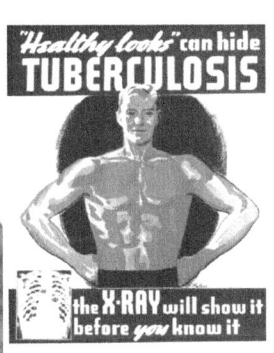

Miliary nodules from TB   *Roentgen*   *Health promotion poster*

In **1895** Wilhelm Conrad Röntgen discovered X-rays. Suddenly there was a technique that permitted the screening of the population: The chest Xray.

Over the last quarter of the 19th century the death rate from TB had been progressively falling. The common populace had begun to get the message that TB was infective and instead of idolising people with the condition they were behaving more like the people of Palma who turned away poor Chopin.

Detection and isolation became the norm. Surgical treatment of the affected patients had a considerable measure of success. Pulmonary tuberculosis (phthisis) occurs mainly in the apices as the bug prefers well ventilated lung. Collapse of the affected part allowed the body's own defences to take over and destroy the tubercle. Unfortunately TB might flare up at a later date if the immune defences were low but at last some amelioration was possible.

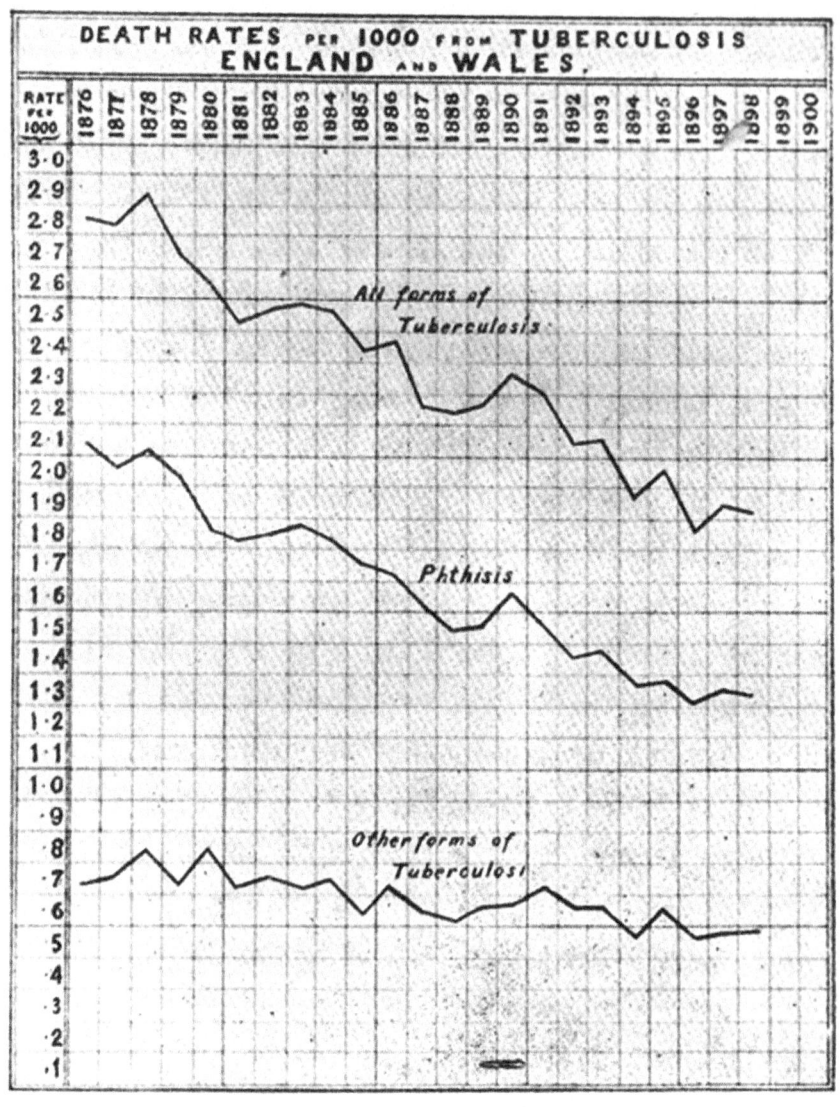

The fall in the death rates per 1000 from Tuberculosis 1876-1900 [8]

The chart above is from a paper in the Bristol Medico-Chirurgical Journal from 1901 showing the progressive fall in the death rate.

Other forms of tuberculosis include Pott's Disease (spinal TB as discussed earlier) and scrofula. The latter is also known as the King's Evil.

The King's Evil

The King's Evil is a strange title for a disease. It does not, however, refer to a mad and evil monarch, such as Vlad the Impaler, but to a disease: scrofula.

"*Scrofula,*" from Latin "*scrofa*" meaning "*sow,*" and the synonymous "*struma*" and "*escrouelles*" derive from the common appearance of the patient's enlarged neck. This is supposed to have caused the sufferers to have a pig-like appearance. "*Morbus regius*", "*mal de roi*" and the "*King's Evil*" are also synonyms for scrofula.

Scrofula is an enlargement of the cervical lymph nodes due to Tuberculosis or due to non-tuberculous (atypical) mycobacteria.

There are many possible causes of the appearances of Scrofula other than TB, such as cervical lymphadenopathy of any cause, extension of a primary neoplasm (e.g. lung cancer), goitre and cysts.

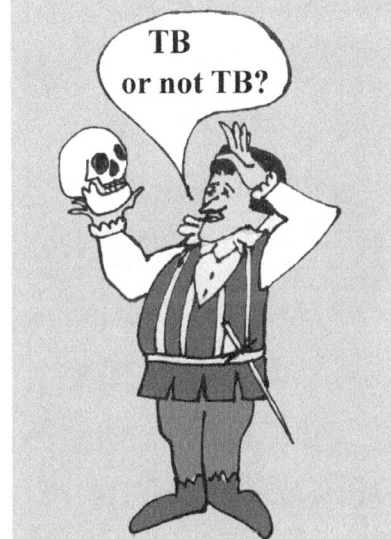

Today the diagnosis can be made by diagnostic imaging and fine needle aspiration cytology and culture. The cause of scrofula was, however, unknown until the late 19th century. The connection with tuberculosis in its other manifestations had not been made.

Ancient Egyptians treated scrofula with surgery and dressings. Hippocrates advocated confinement to the temples of rest, praying, drinking milk, dieting and avoidance of extreme weather. Galen added gargles. The Chinese treatment was acupuncture.

In addition to these relatively practical approaches for many centuries it was believed that scrofula could be cured by the Royal Touch and the giving of a coin by the King to the sufferer. Hence it was called the King's Evil. The Emperor Vespasian started the tradition of 'touch-pieces'. He is said to have given coins to the sick at a ceremony known as the 'touching.' After the Romans had left England science went into abeyance. Anglo-Saxon medicine consisted of herbal remedies, leeches and amulets. The latter sometimes included coins…. Not usually their own coins which were very

Bronze coin of Constantius Gallus showing a Soldier spearing a fallen horseman. (diameter shown x 1.5)

crude but more interesting coins from the late Roman period....such as those showing a soldier spearing a fallen horseman!

Legend has it that the healing power of the Kings of England and France dates back to King Clovis of France who was given this gift by St Remy in 496 AD.

The gift of healing through touch, accompanied by the sign of the cross, is next mentioned in the reign of Robert the Pious (970-1031), second Capetian king, and touching specifically for scrofula is affirmed in the reign of his grandson Philip I (1060-1108).

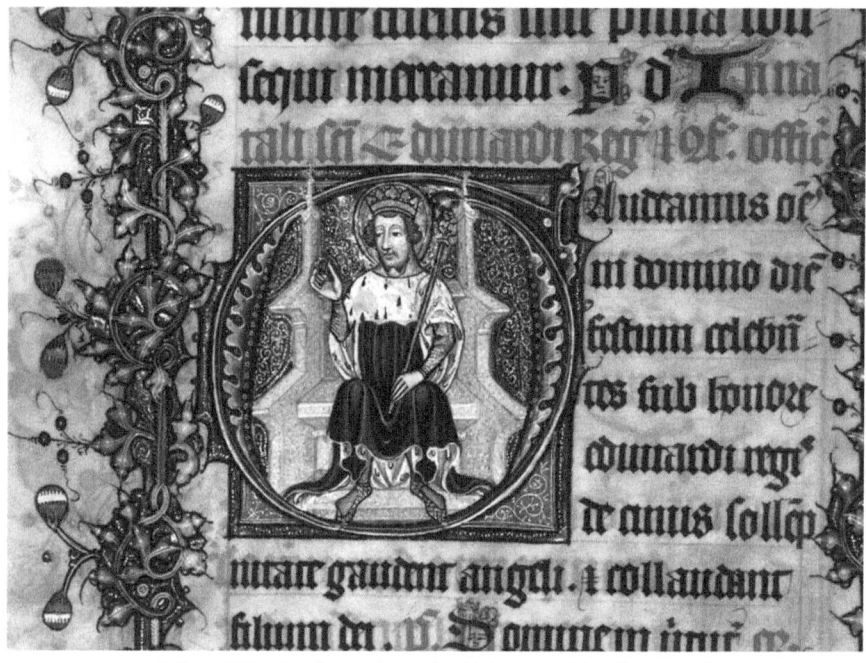

Edward the Confessor from the Litlyngton Missal 1383 AD
With permission (Copyright: Dean and Chapter of Westminster)).

The gift of healing is said to have first manifested itself in England in the hands of Edward the Confessor (born 1003, died 1066).

The kings and queens of England continued to touch patients and give a coin (called an Angel) to magically cure scrofula up until the civil war when Cromwell stopped the practice. Charles II restarted the touching ceremony and in his reign touched nearly 100,000 patients, giving each a gold coin, now called a touch piece rather than an Angel as the latter coin had gone out of usage. The image on it is of the Archangel Michael killing a dragon, symbolic of the devil, and this image is strikingly similar to the Roman coin of the soldier spearing the horseman.

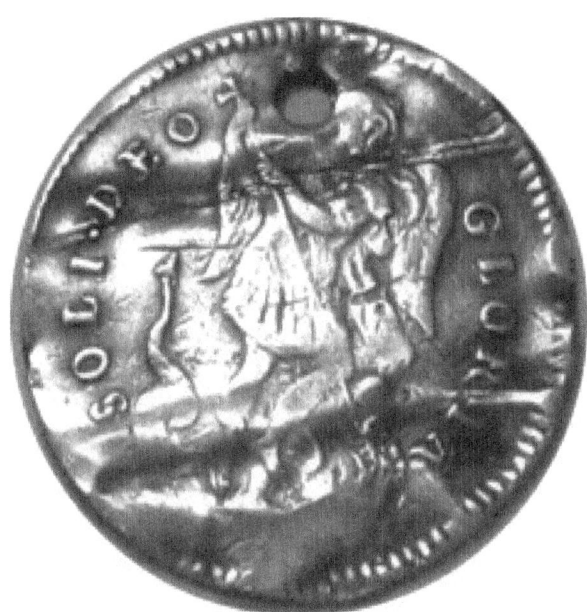

James II gold touchpiece showing Archangel Michael killing a dragon (diameter x 3)

This similarity has not previously been noted by numismatists and the angel design presumably evolved from the earlier talismanic coin. (See above).

James II continued the practice even after he was exiled. His son touched as James III, Bonny Prince Charlie touched as Charles III and his brother, Cardinal Henry, touched as Henry IX. William and Mary stopped the ceremony but it was restarted by Queen Anne, who was the last reigning monarch do to so.

Scrofula and Touching by Royalty in the South West

Marie Trevelyan, in her book *Glimpses of Welsh Life and Character* states : *In 1666 we find a housewife noting…* "*Heard this day how a man in Bristol came home cured of the Evil, the King having touched him*" [9]

Queen Anne had no desire to "Touch" but was persuaded to do so by her ministers. She visited Bath on August 29th 1702 and Bristol on September 3rd. Playing cards relating to these events do show her touching for the Evil and it is possible that she touched in both places.

Samuel Werenfels wrote in his *Dissertation Upon Superstition in Natural Things* in 1749 about a Bristol labourer named Christopher Lovel…. "*afflicted by the King's Evil set out from England in quest of relief. He applied to a certain, nameless, hereditary, unanointed Prince. He succeeded in his wishes, was miraculously cured returned home, relaps'd and died of the Struma at last.*"

The King's Healing Touch

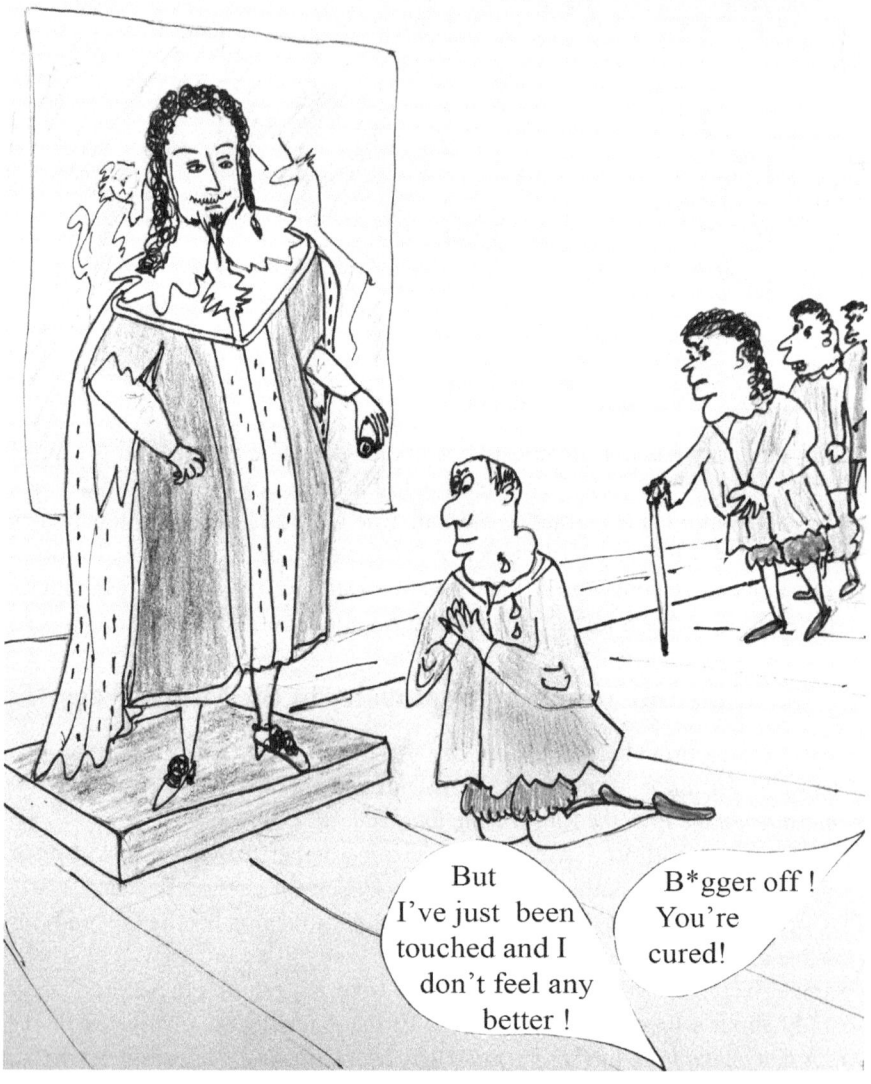

The "Touching" ceremony was important propaganda for the King establishing and promoting his God-given right to rule. (This cartoon first appeared in Fake News)

Quackery

When the touching ceremony was stopped, as in the times of Oliver Cromwell, under William and Mary and after Queen Anne, other forms of 'treatment' would appear and become popular. Thus faith healers would try their luck and various spas were promoted for their healing waters, including the healing of scrofula.

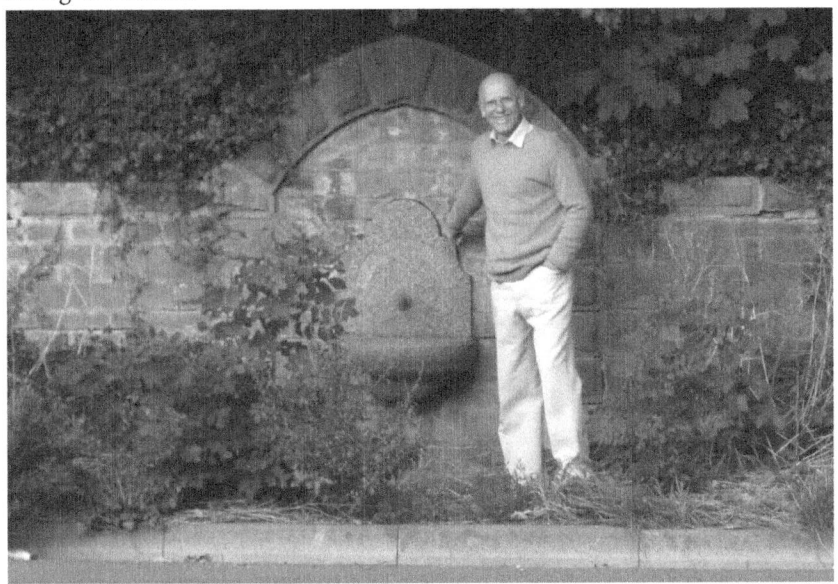

Professor Paul Goddard standing by the fountain on the Portway, Bristol fed by one of the Hotwells Springs

Pigot's Directory of Gloucestershire [10], 1830 tells us: "*The Hotwells are situated about one mile and a half westward from Bristol in the parish of Clifton.
The salutary spring rises near the bottom of the cliff, and so copious as to discharge 60 gallons in a minute. The water is warm as milk, and like those of Bath, famous for the cure of stone and gravel, diarrhoea, diabetes, King's evil, scrofula and cancers.*"

A second hot spring was discovered in Hotwells further down river. This was also promoted as a treatment for Tuberculosis and when John Wesley in 1754 developed "Galloping Consumption" he tried the waters of both wells and preferred the new well. It now feeds a drinking fountain adjacent to the Portway. Touching for scrofula may have made the patient acceptable in society but it did not cure the disease. In fact, by making a contagious patient sociable it almost undoubtedly spread what it set out to cure and the incidence of the disease increased. Mistaken ideas are dangerous particularly when they are irrational cures for infectious diseases.

Bad Habits

Living with multiple people in one room was commonplace in the United Kingdom until well into the 20th century. Nowadays there are UK laws that prohibit overcrowding ...for example your home is overcrowded by law if: *two people of a different sex aged 10 or over have to sleep in the same room. The rule doesn't apply to couples who share a room. Children under 10 aren't counted.* [11]
Spitting is a bad habit and I remember a campaign in the Superman comics in the 1950s encouraging people to not spit in public and also to avoid using a communal cup when drinking from a water fountain.

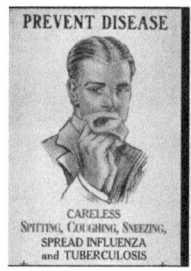
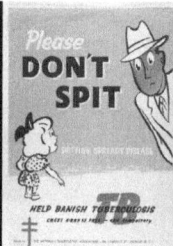
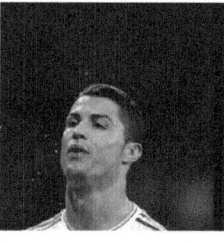
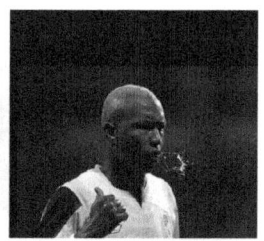

Spitting was banned or heavily discouraged and became unusual behaviour by the 1960s. Unfortunately our sportsmen have brought the habit back into the public's eye. Recently, due to the SARS 2 COVID-19 pandemic the sports authorities have been trying to persuade the players to stop spitting. So some good may come out of this bad time.

Vaccines and Drugs

The BCG vaccine (Bacillus Calmette-Guerin)was first used in 1921 and has been used ever since. It was developed from an originally virulent strain of M.tuberculosis which was cultured on glycerine potato medium. This took thirteen years from 1908 to 1921 by which time it had become avirulent![12]
Just think ...thirteen years of culturing TB on a potato medium!!
The first antibiotics were not effective against TB but in 1943 Albert Schatz discovered Streptomycin (his boss, Waksman, took the credit). Streptomycin was a game changer. Treatment of tuberculosis now is by triple chemotherapy, choosing from Isoniazid, Rifampicin, Pyrazinamide and Ethambutol.

Personal Experiences of Tuberculosis

When I was very young in the 1950s some good friends of the family lived just down the road. Their mother helped my mum by doing some cleaning and their father, Uncle Ray, was a lovely man but very quiet and unassuming. My mother told me that the reason he was so quiet and could not work hard was because he was suffering from TB of the lungs. He never complained and remained cheerful. We continued to be good friends with the family for many years but in the late 1960s Uncle Ray sadly died from his disease when only in his forties. This was the first victim of tuberculosis that I actually knew in person but certainly not the last.

My elder sister tested positive on the Heaf test * and was never vaccinated with BCG. She believed that she had been exposed to tuberculosis from visiting Uncle Ray in the 1950s.

Recently a German friend told us that in the early 1950s she had tested positive and chest X-ray showed enlarged hilar nodes. She was sent to an isolation hospital for six months but was then allowed home as the disease had not progressed to 'open tuberculosis' .... it did not affect her lungs and she was not deemed an infection risk. Her two cousins were not so lucky and were both sent to sanitaria in the Alps for three years.

In 1977 I worked as a senior house officer in chest medicine in London and I saw patients dying from tuberculosis even though we had triple therapy. The most horrifying aspect was the way in which the sufferer may suddenly cough up huge amounts of blood and nearly exsanguinate before your eyes.

Just before I retired early from the NHS a colleague of mine, a respiratory physician, was admitted to hospital with chest complications with the eventual diagnosis of TB just before he died from the condition. It is highly probable, although impossible to prove, that he caught the infection from one of his patients.

Doctors and nurses have been dying from the COVID-19 infection and the public have been applauding their heroism. But doctors, nurses and carers of all sorts have always put their health on the line when looking after patients. Infectious diseases are obviously contagious and the carers are more likely to catch the disease than any one else. Whilst they take all due care and do take preventative measures they are also very frequently the last to complain and that can be their undoing.

---

* The Heaf test was a diagnostic test for previous exposure to TB. It used a spring loaded gun with six needles in a circle to inject the testing serum into the skin of the forearm. I can still just see the scar from my own test which was over 60 years ago. I can also see the scar on my left upper arm from the BCG innoculation.

I applaud all the workers in the NHS and in the caring community, now and in the past. The medals and the knighthoods go to the sportsmen, the businessmen who donate to the political parties, to the lawyers, politicians and the civil servants. But the people who deserve the honours are the carers.

References

1. The history of tuberculosis: Thomas M. Daniel Respiratory Medicine vol 100 issue 11 p1862-1870
2. Daniel VS and Daniel TM Old Testament Biblical References to Tuberculosis Clinical Infectious Disease Vol 29 issue 6 1999 1557-1558
3. Leviticus 26:16 KJV Holy Bible
4. Deuteronomy 28:22 KJV Holy Bible
5. A Curious Case of Backache MacKinnon JC, Goddard PR Clinical MRI Vol 1 pp29-30 1991
6. The proofs of the existence of a phthisical contagion R Singelton Smith, Bristol Medico-Chirugical Journal July 1883
7. https://en.wikipedia.org/wiki/Robert_Koch
8. Tuberculosis statistics and other preventable disease WH Symons Bristol Medico-Chirugical Journal 19,7. 1901
9. Marie Trevelyan, Glimpses of Welsh Life and Character (Publisher: Carpenter Press Date Published: 2008)
10. Pigot's Directory of Gloucestershire, 1830
11. https://england.shelter.org.uk/housing_advice/repairs/check_if_your_home_is_overcrowded_by_law
12. https://en.wikipedia.org/wiki/BCG_vaccine

Bibliography

- *The History of Medicine, Money and Politics* by Paul R Goddard, Clinical Press Ltd. 2008 ISBN 978-1-85457-050-5
- *Fake News* by Paul R Goddard, Clinical Press Ltd. 2018 ISBN 978-1-85457-0963

Chapter 6
Killer Viruses: Influenza and Polio

Influenza

Two infections that scared me when I was a child in the 1950s were influenza and poliomyelitis. We heard talk of the influenza epidemic of 1918 which had killed more people than World War 1 and in 1957 we had our own epidemic. The 1918 epidemic infected 500 million and killed 50 - 100 million. The disease is thought to have originated in China (not Spain!) and was as prevalent in France, Germany and England as it was in Spain. The wartime clampdown on news meant that the deaths amongst our troops and the Germans were not broadcast and only the progression of disease in Spain, a neutral country, was mentioned in the newspapers.

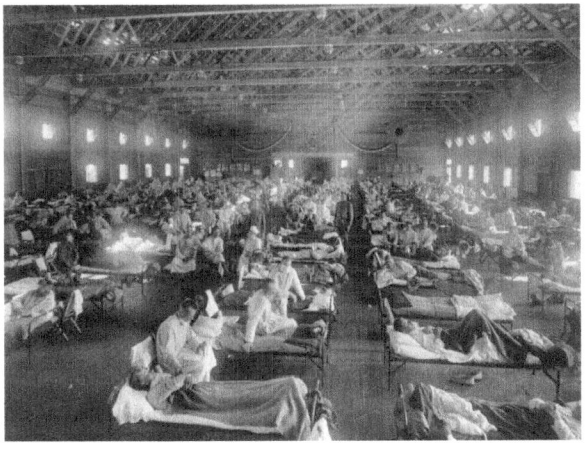

Soldiers from Fort Riley. Kansas, ill with Spanish Flu (H1N1 influenza) [1]

The flu, which killed healthy young adults, may have been brought to Europe by Chinese workers. They had been employed to clear up the battlefields of WW1. It has been suggested that other infections such as tuberculosis or haemophilus influenzae may have been partly to blame for the death toll[2]. We usually expect a viral infection to protect you from an immediate second infection due to the stimulation of interferon but the Spanish Flu did not protect people.

In fact *"In community acquired pneumonia mixed infections occur in up to 27% of cases"*. [3] Pneumonia was probably the most common cause of death. Forms of the tubercle (TB) without cell walls (the L-form) may have been partly to blame.

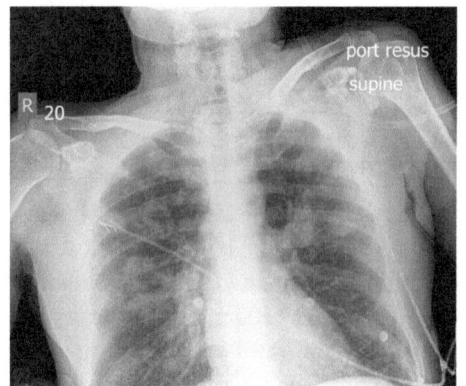 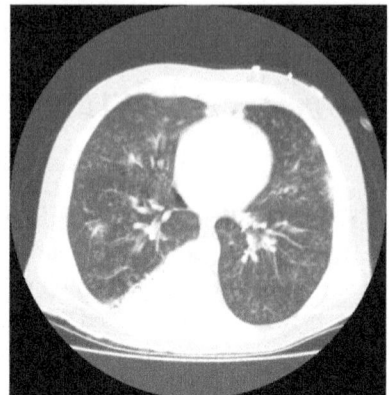

Influenza viral pneumonia on Chest Xray and CT scan
(Courtesy of Dr Judy Holt)

There have been pandemics of influenza on several occasions over the past one hundred and thirty years:

Pandemics

Name	Date	World population Billions	Subtype	Infected	Deaths worldwide	Pandemic severity
Flu epidemic	1889-90	1.53	H3N8 or H2N2	c.600 million	1 million	2
Spanish Flu	1918-1920	1.8	H1N1	c.500 million	50-100 million	5
Asian flu	1957-58	2.9	H2N2	>500 million	1-4 million	2
Hong Kong flu	1968-69	3.53	H3N2	>500 million	1-4 million	2
Mexican swine flu	2009-2010	6.85	H1N1/09	0.7-1.4 billion	150,000-600,000	1

The chart above was adapted from Wikipedia[4]. The typical seasonal flu kills as many as the "Mexican Swine flu" of 2009 every year. Some patients who recovered from the Spanish Flu had late sequelae such as tachycardia or neurological pathology.[5]

Personal Recollections

Everybody has recollections of "The Flu" affecting themselves and their relatives. Here are a few from my own family specifically related to the pandemics:

- 'My grandmother suffered from the Spanish Flu in 1920 and this was followed by a bout of encephalitis. Thirty years later she developed post-encephalitic Parkinson's Disease with severe intention tremor. This improved dramatically with L-Dopa but, sadly, that improvement soon wore off. She survived until 1980, dying at the age of eighty-six.'
- 'I remember at the age of seven (1957) going down with the flu. I knew I was very ill because they made a bed up for me in the sitting room and watched over me, something that only happened when we had a dire condition. I had a very high temperature and became delirious. I remember hallucinations of the floor becoming covered in water and the level rising so that it was up to the bedding. I asked my father why the water was there. He said that there was no water and it instantly disappeared. Another hallucination came about because I had been reading my favourite comic, The Eagle. Just like Dan Dare I was in a very small spaceship and a huge robotic spaceship was trying to grab me. It turned out that the grabbing robot was in fact my father who was trying to cuddle me.'

My wife remembers the effect on her school of the 1968-69 pandemic.

- 'The school was basically shut down. Half of the dormitories were made into an infirmary and the beds were filled with suffering children. As the beds filled up the fit children had to find other beds to sleep in, their own having been commandeered. I was lucky enough to avoid the flu and rather enjoyed long hikes as classes were curtailed. None of the children died and we were sent home early for an extended half-term.'
- 'My father-in-law was a very fit man, playing tennis or badminton most days of the week and singing in choirs until he was eighty-nine. He developed pneumonia in 2009 during the Swine Flu epidemic. He never really recovered his full fitness and he suffered from asthma from then on, a condition he had not previously suffered from. It took away his confidence. He gave up driving and the sports, entering a nursing home in 2012 but kept going with the help of the excellent nursing at the home until 2017. The coughing and breathlessness plagued him until he died.'

Man Flu

For some time there has been a running joke that men complain more about the symptoms of colds and the flu than their counterpart female. This is described in disparaging terms as "Man Flu," and is something which is thought to exist only in the minds of the whinging men. But a report in the BMJ, quoted in the Guardian in 2017, supports the idea that men do indeed suffer more from common colds and from influenza. Research from the US showed men had a higher risk of ending up in hospital from the seasonal flu than did women and that they did not curtail their activities as much as women when they had minor respiratory illnesses. [6] My cartoon reinforces the stereotype as it is definitely funnier.

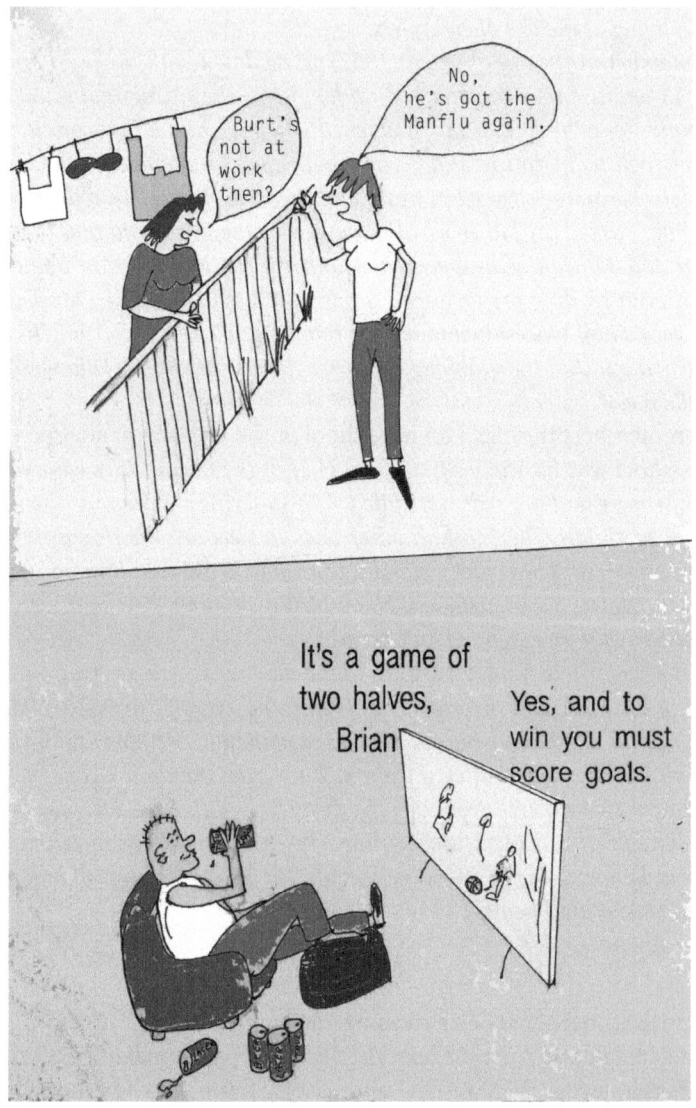

Some of the famous people who died from Influenza [7]

Dimitri Mendeleev 1834-1907 Formulator of the periodic table. Using his table he correctly predicted the existence and atomic weights of at least eight elements now called Scandium, Gallium, Germanium, Technetium, Rhenium, Polonium, Francium and Protactinium.

Reihen	Gruppo I. — R^2O	Gruppo II. — RO	Gruppo III. — R^2O^3	Gruppo IV. RH^4 RO^2	Gruppo V. RH^3 R^2O^5	Gruppo VI. RH^2 RO^3	Gruppo VII. RH R^2O^7	Gruppo VIII. — RO^4
1	H=1							
2	Li=7	Be=9,4	B=11	C=12	N=14	O=16	F=19	
3	Na=23	Mg=24	Al=27,3	Si=28	P=31	S=32	Cl=35,5	
4	K=39	Ca=40	—=44	Ti=48	V=51	Cr=52	Mn=55	Fe=56, Co=59, Ni=59, Cu=63.
5	(Cu=63)	Zn=65	—=68	—=72	As=75	Se=78	Br=80	
6	Rb=85	Sr=87	?Yt=88	Zr=90	Nb=94	Mo=96	—=100	Ru=104, Rh=104, Pd=106, Ag=108.
7	(Ag=108)	Cd=112	In=113	Sn=118	Sb=122	Te=125	J=127	
8	Cs=133	Ba=137	?Di=138	?Ce=140	—	—	—	— — — —
9	(—)	—	—	—	—	—	—	
10	—	—	?Er=178	?La=180	Ta=182	W=184	—	Os=195, Ir=197, Pt=198, Au=199.
11	(Au=199)	Hg=200	Tl=204	Pb=207	Bi=208	—	—	
12	—	—	—	Th=231	—	U=240	—	— — — —

Mendeleev's table of 1871 [8]

One of my favourite songs is Tom Lehrer's listing of the Chemical Elements to an old Gilbert and Sullivan tune. You can find it on Youtube.[9]

Other famous people who died from the Flu

Princess Louise Margaret of Prussia 1860-1917 Duchess of Connaught and Strathearn. Viceregal Consort of Canada.
Harold A Lockwood 1887-1918 Actor, director and producer of silent films
Lord Edward Cecil 1867-1918 Eglish soldier and British Army reformer.
Phoebe Hearst 1842-1919 Mother of William Randolph Hearst
Tallulah Bankhead 1902-1968 Actress
Bertrand Russell 1872-1970 logician, philosopher, historian and British aristocrat.
Trevor Howard 1913-1988 Actor

Poliomyelitis (Infantile Paralysis)

The visible result of the infection was the reason that polio was so scary in the 1950s. Children were seen hobbling around the school playgrounds with calipers on their poor paralysed legs. My godfather, a tall strong man, had a pronounced limp and one withered leg. I questioned my parents about this and the reply came in one word: Polio!

The fittest young people seemed to be the worst affected and anybody who tried to exercise when they had started the disease risked paralysing the very muscles they were exercising. Polio was a dreaded disease, some people became so paralysed by it that they only survived if put inside a breathing apparatus known colloquially as an iron lung.

I was born in 1950 and I was lucky. My generation had the vaccines and the epidemics, which had been affecting the developed world for decades, were finally stopped. The first vaccine I had was the killed variety that had to be injected. I preferred the follow-up vaccines which were the live attenuated variety administered orally on a sugar cube!

The received wisdom is that polio had become a problem in the 20th century because of our excessive cleanliness. The virus had always been around but the bad sequelae only occurred in any number if you missed out on the mild gastro-intestinal upset that polio caused in infancy.

But poliomyelitis paralysis was not in fact a new phenomenon. Egyptian art depicts people with typical withered limbs. Until recently it was possible to see

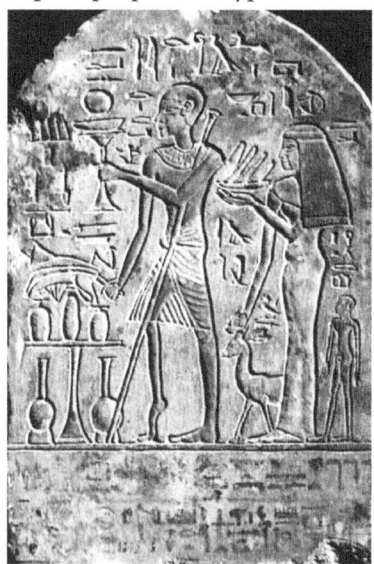

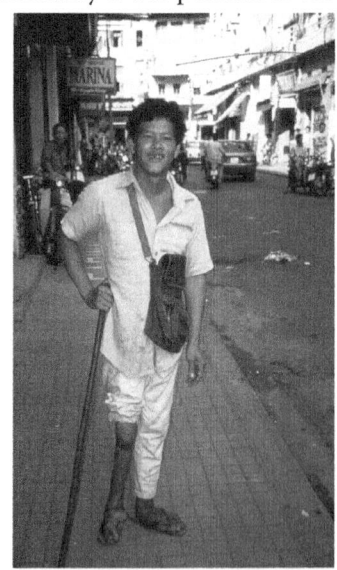

*Left
Egyptian Stele showing a man with a withered right leg*

*Right
Victim of polio with similar atrophy and paralysis of his right leg*

people with similar atrophied limbs in the street in places such as Bangladesh and Pakistan, and in sub-Saharan Africa.

In 1974 in Nigeria I saw a patient with the resident medical officer, Dr. Tom Garrett. The patient had quadriplegia but normal sensation. He was using his diaphragm to breathe because his intercostal muscles were paralysed. Tom sent him off to the nearby university hospital as he clearly had poliomyelitis and needed to be on a ventilator. We heard later that he had died

Now poliomyelitis has almost been eliminated in the world apart from a few cases due to reversion of the attenuated vacccine into a paralysing form. The last remaining region with wild polio cases are the South Asian countries Afghanistan and Pakistan where the Taliban are preventing polio immunisation, claiming that it is a Western plot to sterilise children. Sadly the incidence has increased again.

Table: Cases of Wild Polio[10]

Year	2015	2016	2017	2018
Afghanistan	19	13	14	21
Pakistan	53	20	8	12

Post-Polio Syndrome

Many years after the orignal, acute infection post-polio syndrome may affect polio survivors. This occurs typically 30-40 years after poliomyelitis . It causes progressive weakness of the muscles that previously were affected by the condition.

Famous survivors who later suffered from Post-Polio Syndrome

Arthur C Clarke
Science fiction writer who calculated the orbit for geo-stationary satellites.

Franklin D Roosevelt
President of the USA. Died ten years to the day before the first successful vaccine was licenced in the USA. But see below.............

Guillain-Barré Syndrome

Franklin D Roosevelt: There is debate as to whether Roosevelt did actually have poliomyelitis. Polio is usually a disease of childhood and he was in his thirties when he became paralysed. An alternative diagnosis is Guillain-Barré syndrome, in which weakness and tingling starts in the peripheries, leading on to paralysis.

Like polio a ventilator may be required as the muscles of respiration can be paralysed. Most patients recover well but paralysis may linger.

It is suggested as a possible alternative diagnosis in Roosevelt's case because it most commonly affects adult men.

The most common infections triggering Guillain-Barré syndrome are campylobacter food poisoning, influenza, cytomegalovirus and Epstein-Barr virus (the cause of glandular fever, infectious mononucleosis). Other viruses, including COVID-19 coronavirus, may trigger the condition as may surgery, trauma and rarely influenza vaccinations or childhood vaccinations.[11] Recently Guillain-Barré syndrome has been listed as a very rare side effect of the Janssen (Johnson and Johnson) COVID-19 vaccine with 108 cases in over twenty-one million recipients of the vaccine and one reported death.[12]

References

1. https://en.wikipedia.org/wiki/SpanishFlu
2. Broxmeyer 2011
3. Bellinghausen et al
4. https://en.wikipedia.org/wiki/influenza_pandemic
5. Post-influenzal tachycardia, J A Birrell in Irritable Heart Bristol Medico-Chirurgical Journal Vol 37
6. Stop accusing men of overreacting - 'man flu' really does exist. https://www.theguardian.com/lifeandstyle/2017/dec/11/stop-accusing-men-of-overreacting-man-flu-really-does-exist-claims-doctor
7. https://www.ranker.com/list/famous-people-who-died-of-influenza/reference
8. The original uploader was Den fjättrade ankan at Swedish Wikipedia. https://en.wikipedia.org/wiki/History_of_the_periodic_table#/media/File:Mendelejevs_periodiska_system_1871.png
9. https://www.youtube.com/watch?v=AcSNOQnsQM
10. https://en.wikipedia.org/wiki/Polio
11. Mayo Clinic, Guillain-Barre syndrome
12. COVID-19 vaccine Janssen: Guillain-Barré syndrome European Medicines Agency

Chapter 7
Syphilis

Syphilis is due to a sexually transmitted spirochaete, *Treponema pallidum*. Although now a sexually transmitted disease it was not always the case that it had to be spread in such an intimate way. As mentioned in Chapter 1 the disease was first encountered in Europe in the late Fifteenth Century when *"a new and terrible disease"* broke out among the soldiers of Charles VIII of France when he invaded Naples in the first of the Italian Wars, and its subsequent impact on the peoples of Europe was devastating .[1]

Where it actually came from in the world is much debated although it was unknown in Europe before the conquistadors invaded the Americas. Recent research by Bruce Rothschild suggests that it originated in the Americas, perhaps as a mutation from the related condition Yaws, and was brought over to Europe by Columbus and company.[2] He based his conclusion on bones showing typical syphilitic changes in the tibia and fibula, clear signs of syphilis at least 800 years and maybe as far back as 1600 years ago. The skeletons examined were from Florida, Ecuador, and three New Mexico populations and they also showed that Yaws was present 6,000 years ago.

Initially syphilis was apparently transmitted by close contact and was rapidly fatal. It evolved into a somewhat more benign form. This is typical for very pathogenic organisms, perhaps because otherwise the disease burns itself out as too many hosts die before they can spread it to another host.

The word "benign" in this context is a relative concept. Without treatment infected people do not beat the disease and, although they may develop a degree of immunity, it never goes away completely but becomes chronic...after the primary chancre (an ulcer on the infected part such as penis, tongue, anus or finger) syphilis progresses to a secondary stage of 'snail track ulcers' of the mouth and throat. In the late or tertiary stage granulomatous lesions develop in the arterial and nervous systems and other parts of the body. This can lead to death from rupture of an aortic aneurysm or general paralysis of the insane. A particular stamping gait is famously typical of Tabes Dorsalis from tertiary syphilis.

I encountered relatively few cases of tertiary syphilis in my medical career but, as a houseman in 1975, I assisted a famous plastic surgeon who was dealing with an old spinster who had lost her nose due to some form of chronic infection and had hidden away due to the shame. We were busy removing the crudding and debris and had passed it over to a microscopist, thinking that we might be dealing with an unusual form of tuberculosis known as Lupus Vulgaris, a now rare condition where a skin infection from TB causes much destruction particularly around the nose and inside of the mouth. There was much consternation when the news came back that the granulomatous material we had been scooping out was in fact the result of active syphilis. This was an example of the tertiary granulomatous stage.

One day in the mid 1980s I arrived to report the X-ray films at a hospital in the centre of Bristol. I had to walk through the waiting room where I could not help but notice a patient lying on the floor and making a strange barking noise like a demented dog. 'Barking mad,' was my unkind interpretation of the event and this predisposed me to look closely at the ascending aorta on the patient's chest radiograph. Sure enough there was calcification in the wall of the aorta which, in that site, was typical of syphilitic aortitis. The poor patient was indeed mad from tertiary syphilis, subsequently proven by blood tests.

Congenital syphilis is transmitted into the foetus via the placenta and can severerly damage or kill the foetus.

Syphilis can be propagated in the laboratory by inoculation of a rabbit or monkey. There is no animal reservoir although it has been found in camels.

Historically due to the success of vaccination against smallpox people did, in the nineteenth century, try to develop a weakened or attenuated form of syphilis to provide immunity. Injecting people with this attenuated form was known as "syphilising". It did not work and only served to infect the recipient with syphilis.

The earliest treatments for syphilis that were at all successful were with heavy metals. Initially mercury was the treatment of choice although its great toxicity and tendency to drive people mad was more than a minor problem. Erlich introduced arsenical compounds in 1910 which were "effective but tedious and not without dangers". [3] Heavy metals have been completely replaced by antibiotic treatment. Historically syphilis has been very sensitive to penicillin but resistance has developed. Other antibiotics may therefore have to be used.

Famous people who are said to have died from Syphilis

- Henry VIII (possible)
- George Washington (unlikely)
- Al Capone (definite)
- Ivan the Terrible (possible)
- Beethoven (possible)
- Stalin (likely)

Lyme Disease

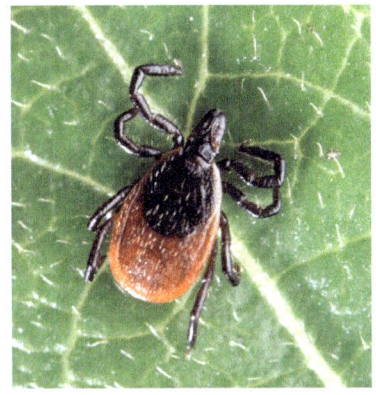

*Deer Tick,
Photo by Scott Bauer.
[Public domain], via
Wikimedia Commons for the
Agricultural Research Service
(ARS).*

Lyme disease, or Lyme borreliosis, is a bacterial infection spread to humans by infected ticks. The bug is known as Borrelia burgdorferi * which is another spiral bacterium or spirochaete. It can be successfully treated with a course of antibiotics if caught in the early stages but if it is not treated in the later stages can cause meningitis, encephalitis, profound weakness, arthritis and cardiac problems.

It has massively increased in prevalence in the UK since the reduction in culling and hunting of deers. The infected ticks can now be found on a variety of other mammals and on grassland.

It has been suggested, controversially but with some compelling evidence, that accidental release of ticks during experiments at Plum Island Animal Disease Center eight miles south of Lyme in Connecticut led to the sudden emergence of the disease and subsequent spread. [5]

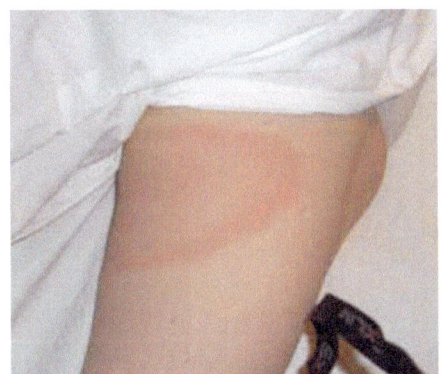

The typical target lesion "bullseye rash" of Lyme Disease [4]

Tests for antibodies are only accurate about 40% of the time and the bullseye rash only occurs in 70-80% of people with Lyme disease.

There is a chronic Lyme condition now known as post-treatment Lyme disease syndrome. The number of people with this may now be as many as two million. [6]

* Note: In Europe the most common organisms causing Lyme disease are Borrelia afzelii and B. garinii.

Leprosy (Hansen's disease)

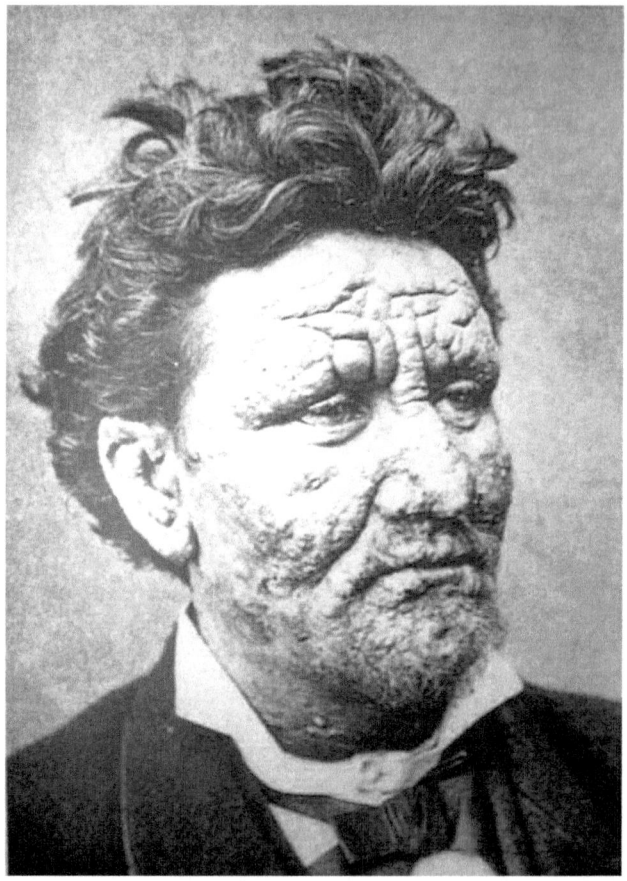

A 24-year-old man with leprosy (1886)
By Pierre Arents [Public domain], via Wikimedia Commons

Leprosy due to Mycobacterium leprae has always captured the imagination because of the horrible later sequelae. Since the antibiotic era and the discovery of Dapsone and Rifampicin the early infection has been treatable but nerve damage cannot be mended. Interestingly 90% to 95% of human beings are said to be immune to leprosy although this is based on relatively poor evidence. [7]

A new strain of Mycobacterium leprae was discovered in 2008 and this may account for some of the variability of leprosy. [8]

Recently it has been reported that red squirrels harbour leprosy [9] and that it is the same strain that was prevalent in Britain in the Middle Ages. Leprosy has always been a disease of poverty and it may be that direct involvement with squirrels (trapping, skinning, eating) spread the disease amongst the poor. Red squirrels have been declining in the UK for centuries, hastened in the past 140 years by competition with the imported grey squirrel but primarily due destruction of the conifer woods and mixed forests that are the red squirrels preferred habitat.

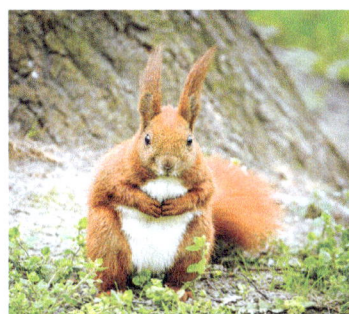 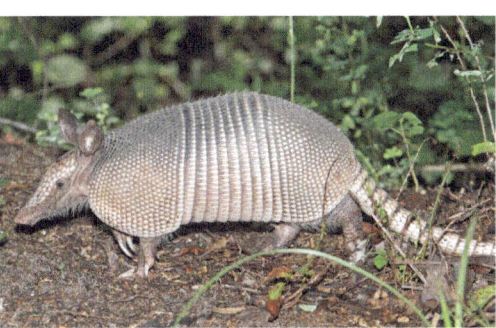

Figure 4 The red squirrel (By hedera.baltica [10])   *Figure 5 A Nine-banded Armadillo in the Green Swamp, central Florida. (Acknowledgement birdphotos .com Reference [11])*

In 1974 during my elective in Nigeria I visited a leper colony and saw active leprosy similar to the photograph from 1886. Imagine my surprise when we were in Rio, Brazil, in 2016 we saw people with the appearance of active leprosy passing us in the street. The highest incidence of leprosy in the world occurs now in India but Brazil also has a very high incidence.

One of the only animals to easily catch and spread leprosy is the armadillo, native to South America and the south of North America. This is reputed to be due to the armadillo's low body temperature. In addition to the red squirrel and the armadillos some other intermediate hosts include mangabey monkeys, rabbits, and mice (on their footpads). The sooty mangabey model of leprosy led to the discovery that rhesus monkeys were more susceptible to leprosy when co-infected with simian immunodeficiency virus (SIV), but that leprosy may play a protective role against acquired immunodeficiency syndrome (AIDS) mortality. [12,13]

My small experience of the treatment of leprosy with Dapsone led me to make a discovery. In 1975 I was working at the Westminster Children's Hospital and we had a patient with severe pustular psoriasis, a condition which looked a bit like leprosy. I suggested we use Dapsone and found that it was very effective. This case was reported at the Royal Society Of Medicine. This was considered to be a completely new use for the drug but I now have found a reference to its use in another single case in 1973.[14]

Sepsis

When bacteria enter the bloodstream they are usually controlled by the body's immune response. There may be a temporary bacteraemia but if this is unchecked it becomes septicaemia, a condition which is now often referred to as sepsis.

Perhaps the most widely publicised example of this is mengingococcal septicaemia which can be a devastating condition leading to rapid death if not recognised. The early signs include tiredness, sudden high fever, severe and persistent headache, neck stiffness, nausea and vomiting, photophobia (discomfort in bright lights), joint pain and drowsiness or confusion.

Untreated the condition leads on to haemorrhage under the skin manifesting as a reddish or purple rash. When a glass is pressed against the rash it does not turn white and this is a very important sign.[15] The condition is a medical emergency which needs treating with antibiotics and intravenous fluids.

Other bacteria can also cause sepsis and the following case report is an example.

Case report: Patient B, a boy aged six years presented with several days history of mild malaise with muscle aches and a purpuric rash for the previous twenty-four hours. The only other member of the family suffering from malaise and muscle ache at that time was B's mother who remarked that the limb pains were very similar to Dengue fever that both she and the patient had caught in Brazil some two years earlier. B's sister and father were not complaining of any similar condition.

On examination the purplish-red rash was present on Patient B's hands, back, buttocks, legs and soles of his feet. On his feet the rash was confluent covering much of the anterior part of the feet. On examination of his mouth he had petechial spots on the posterior part of his palate. There was slight reddening around his mouth and his nares were reddened. The "tumbler test" or "glass test" showed that the rash on his body and limbs did not fade with pressure[15]. Patient B's parents took him to hospital in view of the high possibility of septicaemia. By the time he reached hospital he was bleeding from his nose, which continued for two days, and he was very much more moribund.

Patient B was immediately admitted to the children's ward and put in isolation with his parent. Blood was taken for blood count, urea and electrolytes and

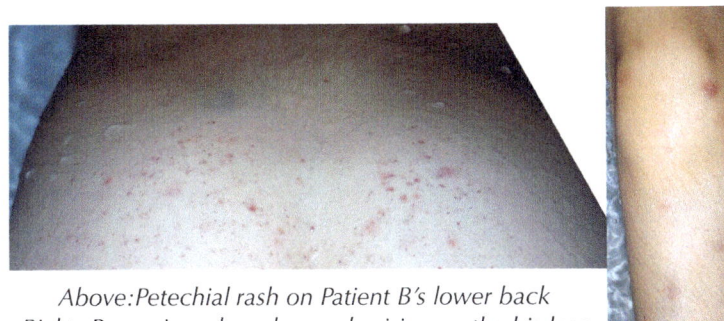

Above: Petechial rash on Patient B's lower back
Right: Purpuric rash and some bruising on the his legs

blood culture. The immediate results showed dehydration and profound thrombocytopenia with the platelet count at one thousand or less (1000 being the lowest level measurable). Viral infection was considered to be highly likely as a cause of the problem. Intravenous cannulation was performed and the patient showed some immediate general improvement with the rehydration but the improvement was not sustained. On day 3, at forty-eight hours, a gram -ve bacillus was reported to have been cultured from the blood and the patient was put on intravenous antibiotics which were changed on day 4 when the full report with sensitivities was obtained. Improvement was then rapid.

The organism cultured was Acinetobacter lwoffii, a gram negative bacillus which is found as a normal skin commensal in 40% of people. Acinetobacter lwoffii is not usually pathogenic and is normally only implicated in patients with immune suppression or severe malaise.

The likelihood is that the sepsis was a secondary infection following a viral disease affecting both patient B and his mother. When a report was received that his two pet rabbits had died it became clear that the rabbits and patient B had been infected with Rabbit Hemorrhagic Virus (v2). This new variant of the Lagovirus, RHDV, was discovered in 2010 [16]. The patient's grandmother, who had been staying with the family, then complained of malaise, muscle ache and some bleeding from her gums which improved without treatment over a week.

Patient B received ten days of IV antibiotics in hospital, followed by two courses of oral antibiotics as an outpatient. He has now made a full recovery.

Caliciviruses exhibit high levels of host switching [17,18] and reports that RHDV(v2) is host specific to rabbits is incorrect. It is postulated, that patient B, his mother and subsequently his grandmother all contracted Rabbit Hemorrhagic Virus (v2) and that patient B was super-infected with the skin commensal which was markedly worsening his prognosis until he received antibiotics.

A. lwoffii [19] is an aerobic gram-negative bacillus occurring as normal flora on the skin and in the orophaynx of between 25 and 40% of the population. It has been identified as the causative organism in urinary tract infections, skin and wound infections, septicaemia, meningitis and gastro-enteritis. However it is usually only pathogenic in immune compromised patients.

Worryingly in Australia the farmers are purposely spreading Rabbit Hemorrhagic Virus (v2) in an attempt to reduce the invasive rabbit population thus mimicking the way that they spread myxomatosis in previous decades. In Britain the wild rabbit population has fallen by 48% in less than twenty years coinciding with the spread of the viruses and vets have issued a warning that pet rabbits should be vaccinated [20]. This case is an example of life-theatening sepsis from a common bacterium in a boy weakened by a zoonotic infection. It is likely that zoonotic infections will become more frequent as human beings increasingly impinge on the animals' habitats and take the creatures for food or pets.

Scarlet Fever

Before the advent of antibiotics and vaccinations childhood illnesses were more common and much more serious. In 1934, for example, 250 children from my home town of Croydon spent Christmas in Croydon Borough Isolation Hospital at Waddon because of an outbreak of Scarlet Fever. Then in 1948, 341 children went to Waddon for the same condition and one hundred out of a total of 2,000 with measles. One thousand children had whooping cough the same year, sixty-four going to hospital and four dying.[22]

Scarlet fever is due to group A streptococcus bacteria. It causes a characteristic rash, sore throat and glandular enlargement and used to be lethal in children. Rheumatic fever can follow which leads to permanent heart problems and also affects the skin, joints and kidneys. Sepsis and pneumonia are other complications of the infection.

Recently the disease has made a comeback reaching a 50 year high with 19,000 cases in England in 2016 [23]

In 1959 my family caught the disease. I was aged nine and slightly unwell but my brother, six, was very ill. He had the full rash, sore throat and glandular enlargement. My elder sister was also ill so the decision was made to pack us off to the Waddon Isolation Hospital mentioned above.

I shared a room with brother Stephen. Our sister was isolated in another part of the building. The room that we shared was austere. Bare, no radio, no television, no books, no games, no pens or pencils and no paper. Nothing to entertain us at all. Everyday Stephen was given a very nasty intramuscular injection of penicillin and I remember the pain he suffered on one occasion when the needle would not penetrate well and the injection had to be repeated. The nurse complained that the needle was blunt and rusty!

The general practitioner who had admitted us visited once, our father visited once a week, each time for a very short period. He was not allowed to bring any books, comics or such like but did once bring some grapes which we thought were the best thing we had ever tasted.

We tried to entertain ourselves talking, counting out loud or in our heads, trying to keep our spirits up but it was miserable.

After three weeks we were allowed home, scarred but alive. I promptly went down with the full-blown scarlet fever and was put on oral penicillin. I refused to return to hospital and was fortunate enough to recover at home over the next three weeks.

I had missed almost a term of my junior school and the day I returned they set an intelligence test. The class had been practicing these but I had no idea what they were and just muddled through. When the results came out my parents were told that I would be very lucky to get through the eleven plus as I was not very bright. Maybe, the teacher said, I would be able to get to the technical college. The fact that I was in the top class and had been fifth in the end of year exams did not seem to matter. There were three classes of 33 to 35 so I was in the top five percent. No, the IQ test was the be all and end all! Luckily they were wrong and the eleven plus the next year did not prove to be too much of a challenge.

The loss of a term's schooling almost derailed my education. The lack of schooling during the past eighteen months due to COVID-19 will affect some children far worse than others and, indeed, far worse than the scarlet fever affected my brother and myself!

References

1. Syphilis - its early history and treatment until penicillin, and the debate on its origins Frith, John, Journal of Military and Veterans Health.Volume 20 Issue 4 (Dec 2012)
2. https://www.discovermagazine.com/health/the-origin-of-syphilis
3. A Short Textbook of Medical Microbiology 1969 Turk and Porter
4. WEMJ Volume 113 No. 1 Article 1 Case Report of Lyme Disease: Lois Tutton BDS WEMJ http://www.bristolmedchi.co.uk/the-west-of-england-medical-journal/wemj-volume-113-no-1-march-2014
5. https://news.nationalgeographic.com/news/2014/02/140228-lyme-disease-borrelia-burgdorferi-deer-tick-science/
6. Once bitten, Chelsea Whyte NewScientist 6 June 2020 pp 40-44
7. http://www.simmins.org/Site2017/wordpress/the-immunity-myth-a-systemic-re-

8. view-of-the-95-percent-immunity-claim-for-leprosy/
9. Am J Clin Pathol. 2008 Dec;130(6):856-64. doi: 10.1309/AJCPP72FJZZRRVMM. A new Mycobacterium species causing diffuse lepromatous leprosy.han XY1, Seo YH, Sizer KC, Schoberle T, May GS, Spencer JS, Li W, Nair RG.
10. Red squirrels carrying medieval strain of human leprosy http://www.telegraph.co.uk/news/2016/11/10/red-squirrels-carrying-medieval-strain-of-human-leprosy-as-peopl/
11. By hedera.baltica from Wrocław, Poland (Squirrel) [CC BY-SA 2.0 (https://creativecommons.org/licenses/by-sa/2.0)], via Wikimedia Commons
12. By http://www.birdphotos.com (Own work) [CC BY 3.0 (http://creativecommons.org/licenses/by/3.0)], via Wikimedia Commons
13. Int J Dermatol. 2008 Jun;47(6):545-50. doi: 10.1111/j.1365-4632.2008.03722.x.
14. The role of the armadillo and sooty mangabey monkey in human leprosy. Hamilton HK1, Levis WR, Martiniuk F, Cabrera A, Wolf J
15. Generalized pustular psoriasis treated with Dapsone. British Journal of Dermatology 1973
16. The glass test: https://www.meningitisnow.org/meningitis-explained/signs-and-symptoms/glass-test/
17. Emergence of a new lagovirus related to Rabbit Haemorrhagic Disease Virus Ghislaine Le Gall-Reculé†, Antonio Lavazza†, Stéphane Marchandeau†, Stéphane Bertagnoli, Françoise Zwingelstein, Patrizia Cavadini, Nicola Martinelli, Guerino Lombardi, Jean-Luc Guérin, Evelyne Lemaitre, Anouk Decors, Samuel Boucher, Bernadette Le Normand and Lorenzo Capucci Veterinary Research201344:81 https://doi.org/10.1186/1297-9716-44-81
18. Shared Human/Rabbit Ligands for Rabbit Hemorrhagic Disease Virus Emerg Infect Dis. 2012 Mar; 18(3): 518–51 Kristina Nyström, Béatrice Le Moullac-Vaidye, Nathalie Ruvoën-Clouet, and Jacques Le Pendu
19. Caliciviridae https://en.wikipedia.org/wiki/Caliciviridae
20. Acinetobacter lwoffii: Bacteremia associated with acute gastroenteritis Nora G. Regalado, Greg Martin, Suresh J. Antony. Travel Medicine and Infectious Disease Volume 7, Issue 5, September 2009, Pages 316-317 https://doi.org/10.1016/j.tmaid.2009.06.001
21. Nature notes, Pet rabbits at risk from lethal virus. Daily Telegraph 23rd May 2018 p31
22. Case Report: Possible cross-over of Rabbit Haemorrhagic Virus (v2) to a young human boy with subsequent near fatal thrombocytopenia and sepsis. PR Goddard**, LM Tutton, JPG Goddard, L Hildebrandt WEMJ Volume 117 No 2 Article 1 June 2018
23. https://www.yourlocalguardian.co.uk/news/67927.heritage/
24. https://www.cbsnews.com/news/scarlet-fever-makes-a-dangerous-comeback/

Chapter 8
Pandemics of Diarrhoea and Dysentery

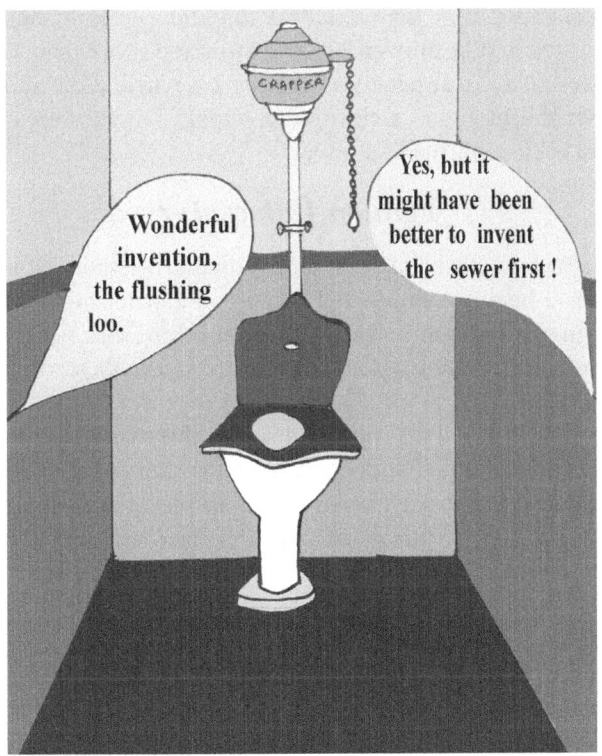

Everybody has suffered from loose bowels on occasion but very few people in the developed countries have encountered Typhoid or Cholera. They both can cause devastating life-threatening diarrhoea and have a similar mode of transmission via contaminated water or contaminated food using the "oro-faecal" route. Unfortunately either of these devastating diseases can occur when the water supply is compromised, something which occurs commonly in times of natural disaster such as earthquakes and hurricanes but is also a major problem when people are displaced by war or revolution.

Cholera and Typhoid

In Haiti a major outbreak of Cholera, caused by the bacterium *Vibrio cholerae*, occurred in 2010 some ten months after a devastating earthquake that killed over 200,000 people and displaced over a million. The start of the outbreak was traced to one of the aid workers who had come into the country to help. There had been no cases for more than a century until the epidemic. Reports in 2020 showed that there had been over 800,000 cases and more than 10,000 deaths since October 2010. Treatment was mainly by rehydration and prevention required re-establishment of a clean water supply. [1] At the time of writing no new cases had been confirmed for a year.

London 19th century

Cholera was a major problem in London in the early to mid 19th century. The water supply was being contaminated because of a major influx of people into the capital. [2] In addition an increasing number of properties had flushing lavatories but the sewers were woefully inadequate, hence the cartoon that opens this chapter. [3]

1854: John Snow realised that the problem was due to micro-organisms in the water supply and in a famous work of epidemiology traced the origins of a major outbreak to a pump in Soho. He removed the handle of the pump and the outbreak diminished. Despite this proof many people would still not believe him. [4]

The Plague of Athens 430BC

During the Peloponnesian Wars of 430BC the Spartans were attacking the city-state of Athens but a terrible plague broke out within the city that was previously unknown to their physicians. In fact the medics were at greater risk of catching it by being in close quarters with the affected patients. Everybody realised that it was very contagious.

The estimates of the number killed in the city range between 75,000 and 100,000, which was about 25% of the population. Pericles, the legendary leader of the Athenians, instigator and builder of the Parthenon, died from the plague.

The symptoms and signs included fever, redness and inflammation of the eyes, sore throats leading to bleeding and bad breath, sneezing, loss of voice, coughing, vomiting, pustules and ulcers on the body, extreme thirst, insomnia and diarrhoea. [5]

The plague was described in great detail by Thucydides and it led to a total breakdown in the rule of law and societal behaviour:[6] *"...the catastrophe was so*

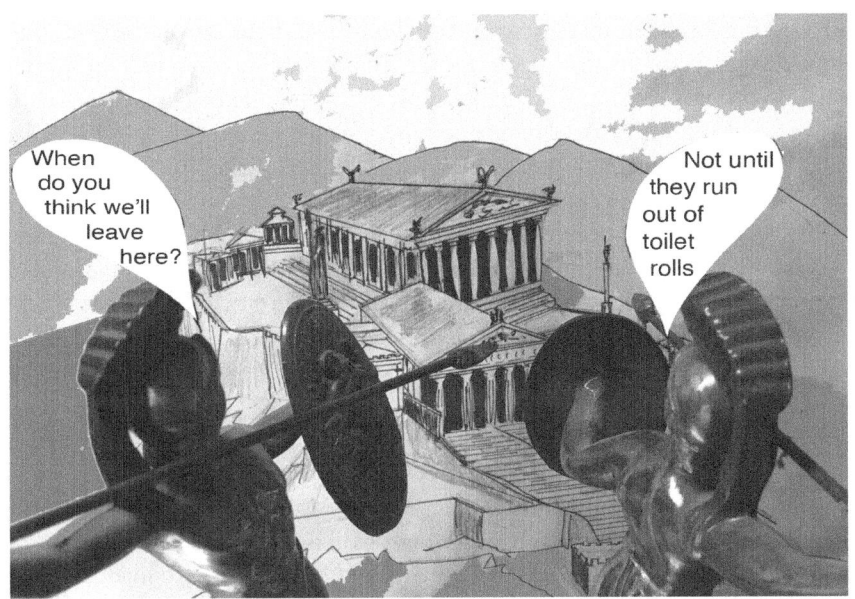

Two Spartan soldiers discuss the Plague of Athens during the Peloponnesian Wars (Apocryphal: Toilet rolls as we know them were not actually invented until 1880). [7]

overwhelming that men, not knowing what would happen next to them, became indifferent to every rule of religion or law."

The written histories were not however, believed until excavations in 1994-95 revealed mass graves and hastily buried human remains from the fifth century BC. Many different pathologies have been suggested but DNA analysis suggested a form of Salmonella, very possibly Typhoid. This has been disputed but is rather convincing. [8]

Bristol: The Unlucky 13

William Budd, who has already popped up in this book in the chapter about tuberculosis, was convinced by **1839** that contaminated water harbouring microorganisms caused typhoid fever. Budd had spent four years in Paris where he was taught an early version of the germ theory

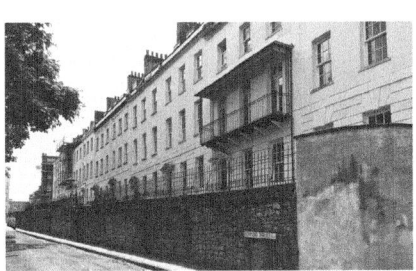

Richmond Terrace

of disease and, on returning to the UK, first to Edinburgh and eventually to Bristol, had dealt with several outbreaks of typhoid fever. In Bristol in 1849 the epidemic was centred among the homes of Richmond Terrace. Of the thirty-four households there were thirteen with at least one case of the fever. The common factor for all of the unlucky thirteen was the use of a well whilst the remaining twenty-one had a different supply of water. Budd recognised the cause and stopped the outbreak. Having attempted, unsuccessfully, to have his germ theory of typhoid published on several occasions over a twenty year period, he eventually succeeded in 1859. [9,10]

Unfortunately many people clung to the view that the problem was due to the miasma or "bad air" and not the result of infection. They thought the problem was due to the gases from swamps and bad drainage, and cited evidence where removal of such miasmic conditions had relieved outbreaks of typhoid, cholera and malaria. Such improvements would also obviously improve the water supply and relieve outbreaks if Budd's theory was correct.

Prince Albert, Queen Vicotria's consort, died in 1861 from chronic gut problems diagnosed at the time as typhoid but this has been questioned more recently as the problems were present for at least two years. This is relatively unusual, but not unheard of for typhoid fever. Other possibilities would include abdominal cancer, ulcerative colitis, Crohn's Disease and tuberculosis (individually, not all at once) but I still accept chronic typhoid as a highly likely diagnosis. Thus disbelief in Budd's theory may have robbed the country of the Queen's consort. It should be noted that the 'lost' River Tyburn is now a sewer running right under Buckingham Palace and when Queen Victoria inherited the building the palace's kitchens kept flooding with sewage.

In **1863** at a convent in Arnos Court, near Bristol, an outbreak of typhoid fever occurred and William Budd was able to establish that this had been brought into the convent by a nun suffering from the condition. The water supply had remained unchanged. Budd advocated the use of disinfectants when dealing with the outbreaks and published this in a series of papers and in his book Typhoid Fever (1873).[11,12]

The Lady with the Bedpan [13]

It is noteworthy that the COVID-19 overflow hospitals set up around the country have all been named Nightingale Hospitals after my favourite medical scientist, the redoubtable Florence Nightingale. Known as the "Lady with the Lamp", she hated that name and stated *"Why don't they call me the Lady with the Bedpan? It would be more accurate."* She was devastated when she realised that more soldiers were dying in her military hospital in the Crimea than were being killed on the battlefield because the medical facilities had been built over defective sewers. Florence Nightingale tried to improve hygiene but was fighting a losing battle. In fact around 16,000 men had died in her hospital from diseases such as cholera, typhus and dysentery compared with just 2,600 in battle and 1,800 directly from their wounds.

To prove her case she developed a great understanding of statistics and the means of demonstrating the data using graphs and pie charts.[14]

In 1860 she established the Nightingale Training School for nurses at St Thomas' Hospital in London. Many nurses were trained in her methods of cleanliness and good nursing, including my own grandmother who was born in 1880 and was, indeed, named Florence after Florence Nightingale. We used to tease my Gran by singing a popular music hall song from 1901:

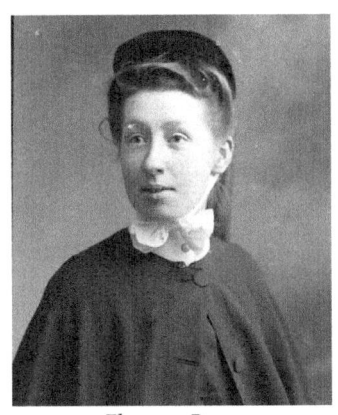

Florence Brown, Nightingale nurse in about 1907

Oh Flo, why do you go
Riding along in your motor car?

We did not realise at the time that this was probably the first automobile song and how striking it was that the person driving was a woman! [15]

Typhoid Mary

The organism that caused typhoid fever was identified in 1879 by Karl Joseph Eberth. It was named *Salmonella* after D. E. Salmon, administrator of the USDA research program.

The concept of an asymptomatic carrier of typhoid fever was not really considered until the organism had been discovered. The first and most famous asymptomatic carrier in the United States of America was Mary Mallon, nicknamed Typhoid Mary. Born in Ireland in 1869, she emigrated to the USA in 1884 and became a cook for a succession of families. In 1906 she, and the family she was working for, became infected with the fever. Mary was only moderately ill and made a good recovery, albeit still hosting the organisms and representing a threat to any person she cooked for. The sanitary engineer suspected that Mary was the cause of the outbreak and looked into her history. She had worked for eight families and seven of them had suffered from typhoid. An outbreak of typhoid infected 3,000 New Yorkers in 1906-1907 and she was probably the main culprit.[16]

She refused to believe that she was in any way to blame and since there was no immunisation against typhoid and treatment was inadequate she represented a very real threat. She tried to elude the health inspectors and police but was eventually quarantined in a cottage. Although one hundred and twenty stool samples proved positive she was eventually allowed back into domestic service as long as she agreed that she would not cook.

She immediately broke the agreement and worked under the pseudonym of Mary Brown as a cook at Sloane Maternity Hospital, infecting twenty-five of the doctors and nurses. Two people died. She was arrested, quarantined permanently and eventually died in 1938, still under strict quarantine.

Arguments still continue about her treatment at the hands of the Health Authorities. [16,17] Apologists claim that she was unfairly treated and that her dangerous status as a carrier was never properly explained to her. In fact they did offer her an operation on her gall bladder and this might have worked if she had accepted it as it is now known that the organism can linger in that site. But she refused and purposely changed her name in order to take on the very work they had warned her about. I disagree with the politically correct apologists. She knew what she was doing and was lucky to not have been incarcerated in a nasty prison for life. I put her in the same category as Daryll Rowe, the UK hairdresser who was convicted of purposely infecting people with AIDS and subsequently jailed for life.[18]

Typhoid in Croydon

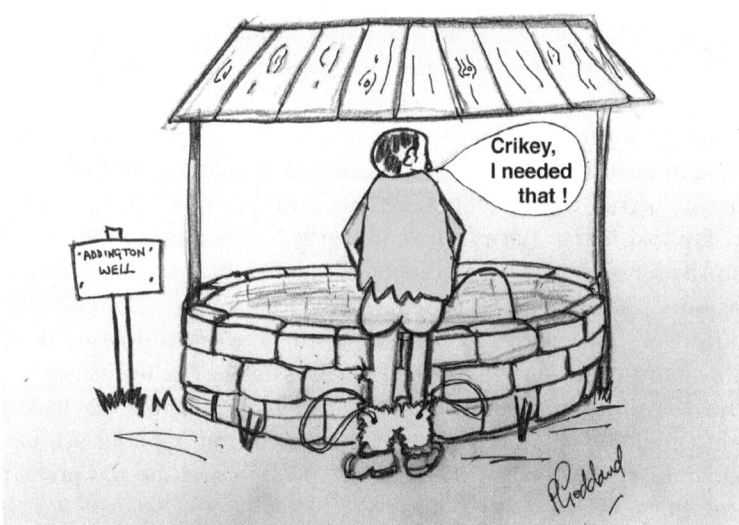

When I was a lad growing up in Croydon the epidemic of Typhoid Fever that had occurred in 1937 was still in the living memory of many of the residents.

I remember my father telling me that it was caused by a typhoid carrier *"weeing in the well."* The story is a bit more complex than that but in essence it is correct.

In the autumn of 1937 there was an outbreak of Typhoid Fever amongst the residents in the south part of the borough. This was initially attributed to shellfish as the first case was of a person who had just returned from France. As the numbers mounted other possibilities such as the milk or watercress were postulated by Croydon's medical officer of health, Oscar Holden. A local resident, Charles Rimington, pointed out that his son had just been taken to the isolation hospital with typhoid fever and that at least two others in the road had the condition. The son later died. The only thing in common was their water supply which came from the Addington Well and pumping station. Holden totally disagreed with the idea, stating that the water was chlorinated and tested. In fact, unbeknownst to him, the testing and chlorination had not occurred whilst the well was being repaired.[19]

The residents formed the South Croydon Typhoid Outbreak Committee (SCTOC) with Rimington as chairman. Eventually Holden was persuaded to enlist the help of Ernest T. Conybeare, the Ministry of Health's expert on typhoid. He mapped out the cases epidemiologically and concluded that the affected water all came from the Addington Well and that a particular workman, a carrier of typhoid, was to blame. It is possible that the workman, who had no idea that he was a carrier but had contracted typhoid fever as a soldier in WW1, did not urinate in the water. The latrines set up for the workmen close to the well did not have satisfactory drainage and could have been the source of contamination.[20] By the end of the year there had been 341 cases and 41 deaths. This was most probably the worst UK typhoid fever outbreak in the 20th century and its origin can be traced back to the First World War.

Typhoid in Aberdeen (1964)

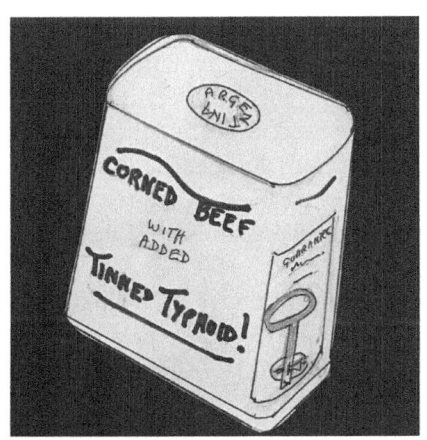

The Croydon epidemic due to the number of fatalities may have been the worst UK typhoid fever outbreak in the 20th century but it certainly was not the last. I have been reminded by Professor Francis Smith of the Aberdeen typhoid outbreak of 1964. This appeared as one single wave with no proven secondary cases. There were 507 cases with three deaths, the mortality rate being so relatively low compared to the Croydon epidemic of 1937 due to the use of the antibiotic

Chloramphenicol, which had been discovered in 1947.

The typhoid occurred due to contaminated tinned corned beef from Argentina. Apparently the tins were being cooled in un-chlorinated river water that was contaminated.

Worryingly thirteen other outbreaks of typhoid between 1929 and 1963 were associated with canned meat including the outbreaks at the Oswestry orthopaedic hospital in 1948, at Pickering in 1954-55 and three outbreaks in 1963 at Harlow, Bedford and South Shields.

Ampicillin could not rival chloramphenicol in efficacy in the Aberdeen cases and there were no cases of marrow aplasia (a rare side-effect of chloramphenicol). There was a reported reluctance to add corticosteroids in non-responsive cases despite evidence that it can be very useful.[21]

Typhus

Typhus is a range of dieases due to Rickettsial organisms [22] and spread by insects.

Typhoid, which is otherwise known as Enteric Fever, was actually named Typh*oid* because of the superficial similarity with Typhus, a condition that people were already familiar with. The mode of transmission and organisms causing the Typhus are completely different from that of Typhoid but symptoms are similar as Typhus also causes fever, headache, shivering, constipation or diarrhoea. In addition weakness of the action of the heart, stupor, coma and death can occur. [21]

Epidemic Typhus is spread by the body louse. It is particularly common during times of war and, as mentioned earlier, was implicated in the deaths of many of the soldiers in the Crimean war.

During the first world war on the Western front typhus fever was conspicuously absent. I have seen it suggested that this was because the men were made to have short hair (thus removing the head louse) and the uniforms had been treated with disinfectants (killing the body louse). The explanation might simply be that they had not brought the disease over with them from the UK but without preventative measures epidemic typhus has been a huge killer in past wars. [23]

Rocky Mountain Spotted Fever is spread by ticks, scrub typhus by mites and endemic (as opposed to epidemic) typhus by fleas. Q fever is also spread by ticks but can be caught from the inhalation of infected material. All are Rickettsial organisms. [22]

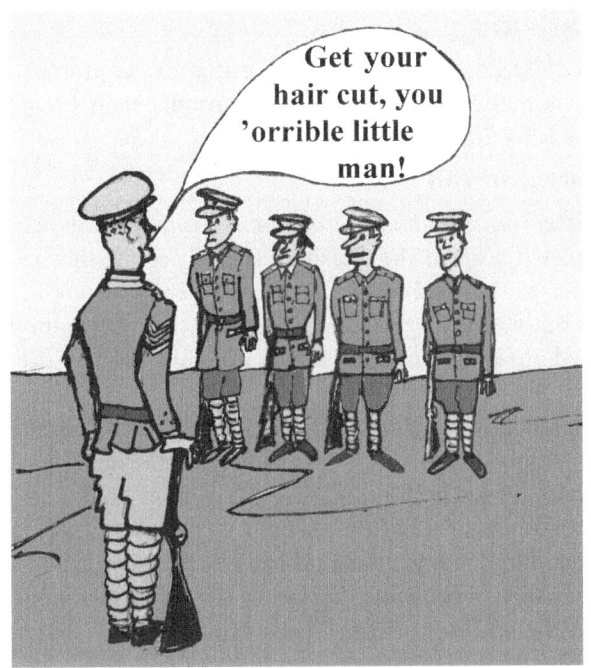

Keeping the hair cut short was necessary to prevent head lice

Dysentery

Bacillary dysentery

Dysentery is an infection and inflammation of the bowel due either to Shigella organisms (Bacillary Dysentery) or to amoeba (Amoebic Dysentery). [24]

When I was in Nigeria in 1974 I suffered from dysentery which, fortunately, must have been bacillary in nature as it responded to sulphonamides. The symptoms were acute onset of diarrhoea, belly ache and mild fever.

I became quite disorientated at one point and was woken up by a nurse who wanted me to see a patient on the wards. Apparently I had been singing a hymn very loudly. I had no recollection of this and had thought I was fast asleep. I still can't sing the hymn without being reminded of the experience.

> *Give me oil in my lamp keep me burning*
> *Give me oil in my lamp, I pray*
> *Give me oil in my lamp keep me burning*
> *Keep me burning till the break of day*

Amoebic Dysentery

This is otherwise known as amoebiasis, is due to the protozoan Entamoeba histolytica. It is harder to treat and more chronic than bacillary dysentery. Metronidazole is the treatment of choice.

Campylobacter enteritis

Campylobacter is a common cause of food poisoning and gave Lois and myself a real fright a few years ago. The diarrhoea was so profuse that we ended up just passing bile per rectum and really felt that we were likely to die. It responded to antibiotics but we were very ill. We probably caught it from poorly cooked chicken served to us in Spain. (Most commonly the enteritis comes from poultry.)

Twenty-three million people fall ill from bad food each year in Europe alone.

The World Health Organisation (WHO) cites campylobacter as one of four key global causes of food poisoning[25]. One in ten people are affected per annum. There are seventeen species and six subspecies. The onset is between one and ten days after eating the contaminated food but usually two to five.

The symptoms are diarrhoea (frequently bloody), abdominal pain, fever, headache, nausea, and/or vomiting. The symptoms typically last 3 to 6 days. Death is rare, usually amongst the very young or the elderly.

Complications, including bacteraemia, hepatitis, pancreatitis, and miscarriage, have been reported with varying degrees of frequency. Post-infection complications may include painful inflammation of the joints which can last for several months and neurological disorders such as Guillain-Barré syndrome, a polio-like form of paralysis (see chapter 6).

Campylobacter species are common in livestock and pets but rarely cause disease. When human beings suffer from Campylobacter enteritis it is another example of zoonotic infection. [25]

Treatment is not generally required, except electrolyte replacement and rehydration. Antimicrobial treatment is recommended in invasive cases (when bacteria invade the intestinal mucosa cells and damage the tissues) or to eliminate the carrier state.

Campylobacter is destroyed by good cooking and avoidance of cross-over between cooked and uncooked food.

Norovirus

Norovirus, the winter vomiting bug, is the commonest cause of diarrhoea and vomiting. It is highly infectious and spreads round in minor epidemics. Washing the hands with soap and water is the best way of preventing spread but alcohol gel does not seem to be effective. Staying at home, resting and drinking plenty of fluids such as water or Dioralyte usually suffice as treament. Seek medical attention if you develop diarrhoea that doesn't go away within several days. Also, call your doctor if you have severe vomiting, bloody stools, stomach pain or dehydration.[26]

References

1. https://www.theguardian.com/global-development/2020/mar/16/it-became-part-of-life-how-haiti-curbed-cholera
2. https://www.sciencemuseum.org.uk/objects-and-stories/medicine/cholera-victorian-london
3. https://www.baus.org.uk/museum/164/the_flush_toilet
4. tps://en.wikipedia.org/wiki/1854_Broad_Street_cholera_outbreak
5. https://en.wikipedia.org/wiki/Plague_of_Athens
6. Thucydides, History of the Peloponnesian War 2.52
7. Toilet Rolls http://www.toiletpaperhistory.net/invented-toilet-paper/who-invented-toilet-paper/
8. Papagrigorakis, Manolis J.; Yapijakis, Christos; Synodinos, Philippos N.; Baziotopoulou-Valavani, Effie (2006). "DNA examination of ancient dental pulp incriminates typhoid fever as a probable cause of the Plague of Athens". International Journal of Infectious Diseases. 10 (3): 206–214. doi:10.1016/j.ijid.2005.09.001. PMID 16412683
9. Budd W. On intestinal fever. Lancet 1859;ii: 4-5, 28-30, 55-6, 80-2
10. Robert Moorhead William Budd and typhoid feverJ R Soc Med. 2002 Nov; 95(11): 561–564
11. Obituary. William Budd. Lancet 1880;i: 148
12. Typhoid Fever: Its Nature, Mode Of Spreading, And Prevention. By William Budd, MD FRS. London: Longmans, Green, and Co, 1873
13. https://www.mirror.co.uk/news/uk-news/florence-nightingale-the-lady-behind-the-lamp-311046
14. https://www.theguardian.com/news/datablog/2010/aug/13/florence-nightingale-graphics
15. https://www.youtube.com/watch?v=ciY4XiRn1qw
16. Mary Mallon (1869-1938) and the history of typhoid fever.Marineli F, Tsoucalas G, Karamanou M, Androutsos G. Ann Gastroenterol. 2013;26(2):132-134.
17. https://en.wikipedia.org/wiki/Mary_Mallon
18. www.independent.co.uk/news/uk/crime/daryll-rowe-hiv-infect-men-hairdresser-brighton-jail-appeal-a8613586.html
19. https://en.wikipedia.org/wiki/Croydon_typhoid_outbreak_of_1937
20. https://www.ncbi.nlm.nih.gov/pmc/articles/PMC2085766/?page=3
21. Aberdeen Typhoid Outbreak of 1964 British Medical Journal 10 Sept 1966 pp 601-602)
22. Typhus: Collins Dictionary of Medicine
23. Typhus: https://www.futuremedicine.com/doi/full/10.2217/fmb-2018-0323
24. Dysentery: Collins Dictionary of Medicine
25. https://www.who.int/news-room/fact-sheets/detail/campylobacter
26. https://www.nhs.uk/conditions/norovirus/

Chapter 9
The AIDS Epidemic

In the early 1980s a mysteriously large number of people developed a previously rare pneumonia with a bug called *Pneumocystis carinii*. This is known as PCP pneumonia. * see note below

I have good reason to remember this bug as in 1975 I was the houseman on a paediatric ward of a famous London teaching hospital and an infant boy came in with pneumonia. The paediatric team assured the worried parents that athough the boy was severely ill he would recover quickly with antibiotics. This was not the case and he went progressively down hill. Eventually the pathogen was discovered, *Pneumocystis carinii*, and he was treated with Co-trimoxazole (Septrin). By this time we had learnt from the many blood samples that the lad was suffering from an unusual immune deficiency syndrome. I believe now that this was a case of congenitally acquired Human Immunodeficiency Virus (HIV) but I have no proof. I had referred the case to the locum senior registrar and had acted in all good faith on his instructions. Together we put the poor child on a ventilator and treated as vigorously as possible, all to no avail. There was an initial slight response to the Septrin*, but then his condition worsened and, to much anguish all round, he very sadly died.

At the subsequent "mortality and morbidity" meeting the senior staff tried to shift the blame on to me. I refused to accept this and pointed out that I had referred the case to my next up in command, that we had given the right treatment and that the poor boy had a peculiar immunity problem. One of the consultants had some fame in immuno-compromised cases and his main grouse was not that the child had died but that I had not informed him and he would have found the case most fascinating.

As noted above just a handful of years later in the 1980s peculiar pulmonary infections started to happen in a disturbingly large number of people. This was an epidemic of PCP pneumonia and it was discovered that all the sufferers had immune deficiency. This condition was dubbed Acquired Immunodeficiency Syndrome or AIDS and the Human Immunodeficiency Virus (HIV) was identified as the cause. Originally it was thought that they were all associated with

---

*Note: *Pneumocystis carinii* is now considered to be a fungus but was previously classified as a protozoan. The name has been changed to *Pneumocystis jirovecii*.
* Septrin, also known as Bactrim and Cotrim, is actually a combination of two drugs: trimethoprim and sulfamethoxazole hence the name co-trimoxazole. It is still the firstline treatment for PCP pneumonia.

Haiti, then that they were all homosexual or drug addicts.

Eventually Dr. Angus Dalgleish pointed out that Slim Disease in Africa was actually Acquired Immune Deficiency Syndrome (AIDS) and that Slim Disease predated the world pandemic.[1]

Kaposi's Sarcoma is another marker of AIDS and before the discovery of AIDS Kaposi's Sarcoma was considered to be very rare except in Ashkenazi Jews. It is caused by a relatively common virus, human herpesvirus 8 (HHV-8) but only causes the sarcoma in immunocompromised people. When I was in Nigeria in 1974 there was an epidemic of Kaposi's Sarcoma. This is now known as endemic African Kaposi's Sarcoma and is classified separately from HIV-related Kaposi's sarcoma but, in fact, many of the sufferers test positive for HIV.[2] African Kaposi's Sarcoma was first described in Africa in the 1890s.

Many people, unknown, famous and infamous, died at the initial outbreak of the disease. There was no quarantining and contact tracing was hampered by the fact that the medical teams in the UK and possibly also elsewhere were not permitted to pass on the information that the patient was infected with HIV and, unlike TB and many other diseases, the condition was not, and is still not, a notifiable disease in the UK.

Eventually in the 1990s triple therapy for AIDS was established.

Weirdly enough I have now heard rumours of people purposely becoming infected so that they can go on therapy and then *"they would not have to worry about the contacts they make with other infected people."*

So the complacency soon returns.

Many people are expecting a vaccine against AIDS to be available soon. In fact the latest vaccine created against AIDS actually made things worse.[3] The vaccinated people became more likely to get the virus so the trials had to be stopped.

Theories regarding the origin of AIDS

There have been many conspiracy theories regarding the origin of AIDS, mostly suggesting that it was purposely propagated by the Americans. These theories have not been found to have any foundation in fact. The virus appears to have originated from the closely related simian immunodeficiency virus (SIV) and passed to humans as a zoonotic disease, perhaps when chimpanzees were eaten as bush meat or kept as pets.

The suggestion that HIV or SIV contaminated the early oral polio vaccines have not been substantiated. Batches of the early vaccine have been tested and no simian viruses or chimpanzee DNA has been found in them although traces of macaque mitochondrial sequences were detected.[4]

It is quite possible that some of the early vaccination programmes in Africa did spread hepatitis and AIDS via multiple usage of the same unsterilised needles.

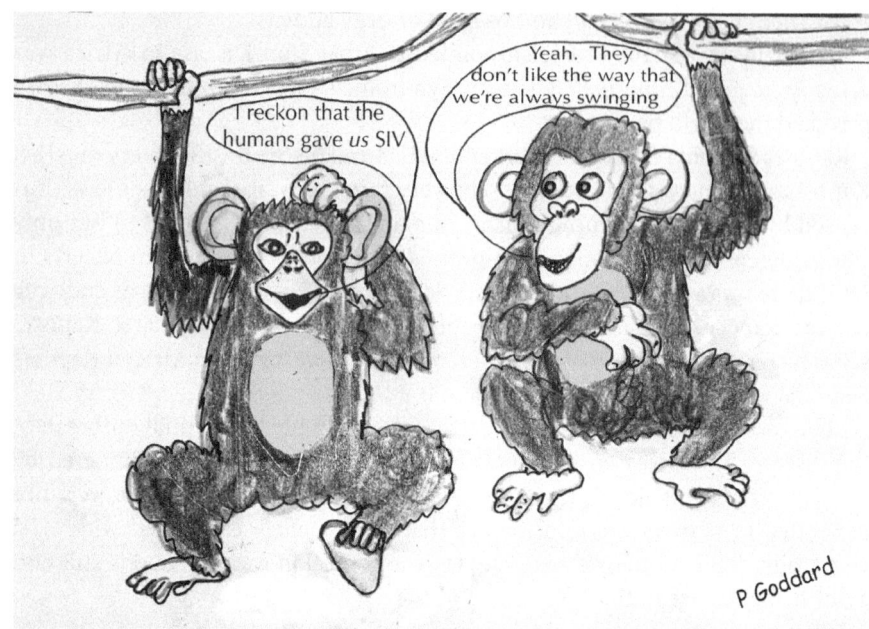

Famous people Who Died From AIDS

As usual in this book this is only an eclectic selection from the numerous people who have died from the condition

Rock Hudson (1925-1985)

Rock Hudson was the first major Hollywood star to die from AIDS. He had been diagnosed with HIV on June 5 1984 but kept his illness and HIV status a secret until his last few months. Hudson was the ultimate leading man so his homosexuality came as a shock to many of his fans. His longtime friend Elizabeth Taylor co-founded the American Foundation for AIDS Research and the Elizabeth Taylor AIDS Foundation.

Freddie Mercury (1946-1991)

Front man for rock band Queen. *Rolling Stone* magazine put him at number 18 on their list of 100 greatest singers.

Arthur Ashe (1943-1993)

Winner of the singles title at Wimbledon. He caught HIV from blood transfusion during heart surgery.

Hepatitis

In 1976 I was working as a senior house officer in the Accident and Emergency Department of a London teaching hospital. One of my colleagues was in a grouchy and depressed mood when my wife picked me up at the end of my shift.

'He's got a very jaundiced-eye view on the world,' she remarked and I looked at him afresh.

He was indeed jaundiced! The poor fellow was subsequently off work for months.

In 1980 I was working as a senior registrar in Bristol. One of the other trainees was from Zimbabwe and supported the Zimbabwe African National Union - Patriotic Front, otherwise known as ZANU-PF. He also was very pessimistic about the world, his mood not improving much even when his party won the election. He returned to Zimbabwe where, for a time, he was minister of health. He also became jaundiced and later died from a malignant liver tumour.

The two doctors had one thing in common. They had both caught viral hepatitis.

Hepatitis is an inflammatory condition of the liver which can be caused by a variety of insults to the organ including drugs and alcohol. More commonly, as in the two cases described, hepatitis is due to a viral infection.

The commonest kinds of viral hepatitis are labelled A, B and C but D and E also exist and other viruses such as cytomegalovirus, Epstein-Barr virus and yellow fever can also cause hepatitis.[5] Liver function studies show that hepatitis, liver inflammation, is also a feature of between 2 and 11% of patients with COVID-19 coronavirus infection.[6]

Hepatitis C was mentioned in chapter 1 as the tenth worst pandemic in the world. Many of the patients with Hepatitis C were infected by medical treatment, vaccinations, blood transfusion etcetera. Others acquired their infection by sexual intercourse, IV drug use or other means. The re-use of syringes was not known to be harmful until the 1980s and were used medically until the discovery of AIDS.

Fortunately there is a curative treatment now available for Hep C: ledipasvir–sofosbuvir. Unfortunately it is expensive and may be rationed, as in the UK on the NHS or not available at all.

If chronic hepatitis is not treated it may lead to fibrosis and hepatocellular carcinoma. In other words, lack of treatment leads to cancer.

Haemorrhagic Viruses:
Filoviridae (Filovirus) Ebola and Marburg

Ebola Virus Disease (EVD) is a rare, deadly disease that is also known as haemorrhagic fever virus. It mostly occurs in Africa causing widespread bleeding from small vessels. It is spread by contaminated body fluids and contact with infected bodies. Strangely the virus can change a person's eye colour. Sufferers from the virus who were thought to be clear of infection have watched with horror as an iris changed from clear blue to a murky green. The virus has been identified in profusion within the eye but with treatment the eyes have returned to their normal colour. The virus has also been found in semen months after the patient had apparently recovered.

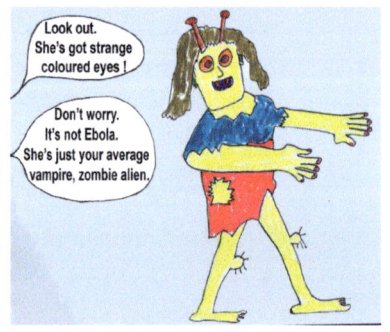

The US Food and Drug Administration (FDA) have approved two specific treaments for Ebola, one a cocktail of three monoclonal antibodies and the other a single monoclonal antibody. Basic intervention with fluids and electrolytes, and treatment of other infections if they occur can improve the chance of survival.

Marburg Virus Disease (MVD) was formerly known as Marburg haemorrhagic fever. It is a rare disease with a mortality rate of about 50%, spread to humans by fruit bats. It was first identified during outbreaks in 1967 occurring simultaneously in Germany and Serbia and these cases were linked with laboratory work using African green monkeys. Transmission can occur from bats or directly, person to person, due to contaminated body fluids and contact with infected bodies. Burial ceremonies that involve direct contact with the cadaver can spread both Ebola and Marburg.

References

1. https://en.wikipedia.org/wiki/Angus_Dalgleish "produced the first link between Slim Disease and HIV infection."
2. https://www.nhsinform.scot/illnesses-and-conditions/cancer/cancer-types-in-adults/kaposis-sarcoma
3. Key HIV trial in South Africa ends because of poor results, The Guardian 3.2.2020
4. https://www.thelancet.com/journals/lancet/article/PIIS0140-6736(00)04536-0/fulltext#article_upsell
5. https://en.wikipedia.org/wiki/Viral_hepatitis
6. Liver injury in COVID-19: management and challenges, Chao Zhang, Lei Shi, Fu-Sheng Wang. https://www.thelancet.com/journals/langas/article/PIIS2468-1253(20)30057-1/fulltext

Chapter 10
It's An Infection
And It's Not What You Think It Is!

In January 2019 an article appeared in New Scientist[1] that made my jaw drop. Not literally, it was still attached firmly to my head, but figuratively. It is an apt description because the article referred to the bug that causes many of the cases of chronic periodontitis*. *Porphyromonas gingivalis, "the keystone pathogen in chronic periodontitis, was identified in the brains of Alzheimer's disease patients."*

For some decades researchers have been pursuing the 'amyloid' theory of Alzheimers. This was based on the demonstration that the brains of patients with the dementia are shot through with abnormal amyloid protein. The identification of Bovine Spongiform Encephalitis (BSE) as a prion disease producing similar appearances in the brains of cows and several other mammals led scientists to the idea that a prion was the cause of Alzheimers.

When I was thirty years old and a senior registrar in radiology I was working with a very kindly consultant radiologist and we started talking about the extraordinary condition known as Kuru. The consultant pulled out some old x-rays of natives from New Guinea. They showed distorted bones and multiple old fractures, a little like chronic alcoholics but much more disturbed. We started writing an article he had always meant to complete detailing the findings of this now almost forgotten condition.

So what was Kuru? A few people with the disease survived until quite recently but the epidemic in Papua New Guinea died down in the 1950s-60s. The native people of the Fore tribe had a habit of cannibalism of their relatives when they died. The story is that the abnormal prion protein was then absorbed into the body and in susceptible people turned otherwise normal proteins in the brain into the entangled mess of amyloid-like proteins. They became progressively ataxic and eventually died with dementia. Apart from those who had late onset due to the long incubation period, the disease disappeared because the Australians came in force in 1960 and forbade the New Guinea tribesmen from undertaking cannibalism in their funeral rites. [4]

1990 and John Selwyn Gummer was Minister of Agriculture, Fisheries and Food whilst cattle were dying from a strange condition much like scrapie, a common condition in sheep. The neurodegenerative condition caused an abnormal gait,

* *Note: periodontitis is a severe gum infection that can cause tooth loss and destroy bone*

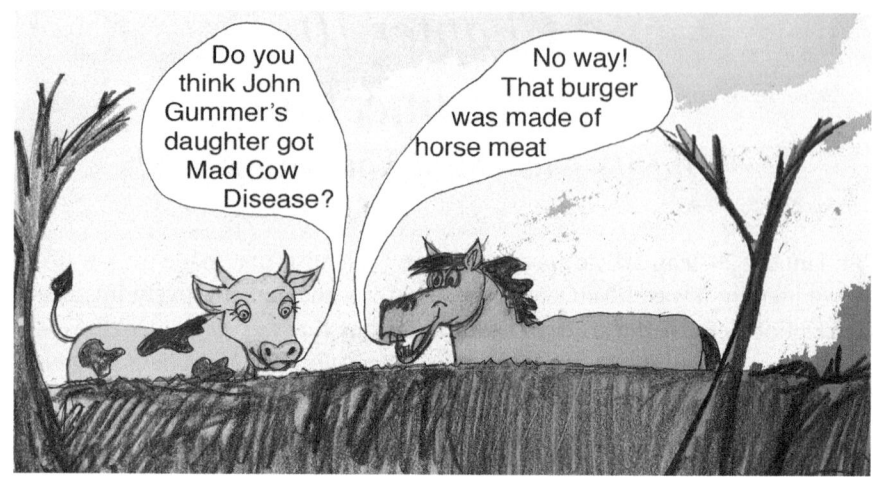

May 16th 1990, three years after BSE had been identified in British cattle, John Gummer famously fed a beef burger to his daughter to demonstrate the safety of British Beef.[2] In 2013 it was discovered that many beef burgers were actually made of horse meat.[3]

aggression and eventually coma and death.[5] It was dubbed *"Mad Cow Disease"* by the media and occurred due to feeding the cows ground-up cattle carcasses in their feedstuff, thus making them into cannibals like the natives of New Guniea.

The agent is an abnormally folding protein (the prion protein) that is not destroyed by cooking and makes similar proteins in the recipient also fold-up abnormally. 180,000 cattle were affected and 4.4 million were slaughtered to prevent the spread.

John Gummer did not believe that this rendered the meat dangerous in any way and to show his confidence he fed a burger to his daughter. She took one bite and pronounced that it was disgusting. He ate the rest and declared that it was wonderful. Both are still alive and did not contract the disease, which was purely luck since the new variant Creutzfeld-Jakob Disease (NVCJD) was later recognised as being one and the same as BSE and you *can* get it by eating meat from an affected cow.

It is not always easy to avoid substances in processed food. The 2013 horse meat scandal was a food industry scandal in Europe in which foods advertised as containing beef actually contained horse meat. The scandal was discovered by DNA analysis of beef burgers in Britain and Ireland. Some contained 100% horse meat.[3]

Similar appearances had been discovered in the brains of people with Alzheimer's disease, a condition that was, at one time, expected to affect as many as one in four persons over eighty years of age. But all the attempts to create drugs that removed the amyloid from the brains of Alzheimer's sufferers have led almost exacty nowhere. Moreover some people had the tangled proteins in their brains but showed no sign of Alzheimer's Dementia. It was a mystery until the report in New Scientist [1] based on work by Dominy.[6]

We have always known that the oral health of Alzheimer's sufferers was bad but this was assumed to be due to the dementia rather than causing it. Association does not prove or even imply causation. Both could be the result of some other factor or just a chance finding. Dominy et al had taken this further and almost completely demonstrated Koch's Postulates with regard to *Porphyromonas gingivalis* (see the chapter on Tuberculosis for the Postulates.) The organism *P. gingivalis* was identified in human brains from Alzheimer's patients. The organism in mice went from an oral infection to the brain where it produced toxins called gingipains. The toxins interfered with tau proteins and caused production of amyloid. Gingipains have also been found in human beings associated with typical Alzheimer's plaques. In lower concentrations they have been found in non-Alzheimer's patients which, rather than being a factor against the *Porphyromonas gingivalis* story, has been cited as supportive since it is known that the plaques can accumulate over a long period of time.

Presently there are attempts to produce and administer blockers for the gingipains but these are still in trials as I write.

Since the *Porphyromonas gingivalis* is found in only 90 to 95% of Alzheimer's it is still possible that the prion story is true in some patients or that the organism and its toxins can set off a prion cascade in some patients.

Whatever the outcome of the *Porphyromonas gingivalis* trials it is clear that gingivitis has terrible sequelae and requires vigorous treatment. Can the infection cause other problems? It appears to be implicated in coronary artery disease, diabetes, stroke and premature births or low-weight babies. Dentists have long believed that gum disease had major sequelae on the general health of patients but, most unfortunately, the artificial split between dentists and doctors has meant historically that oral medicine is relatively neglected and ignored by the medical profession. Moreover the NHS has constantly undermined the position of general dental practitioners and community dentists and, with the lockdowns, dentists haemorrhaged money as they are mostly self-employed and have enormous overheads running practices that were not allowed to function. Many will go bankrupt.

Ironically opticians were in the same sinking boat...and this was 2020. This will come back to bite us and none of us will have 2020 vision!

Conclusion

It is interesting to consider what would happen today if we came across a tribe with cannibalism in their funeral rites. Politically correct pundits might well stop a "colonial power" from banning the rites on the grounds that the native people are entitled to whatever religion and sacred rites they like. They might also point out that the holy communion service could be considered as ritualised pseudo-cannibalism *"This is my body...this is my blood"* [7] and use that to conclude that the Fore funeral rites should not be stopped as it would be hypocritical. If such PC thinking had prevailed in 1960 Kuru would still be prevalent in New Guinea.

What of Alzheimer's disease in the UK? At the current rate of prevalence about a million people are suffering from the condition. This is a little lower than previous projections but still extremely worrying. Perhaps good dental care when the NHS was first set up has reduced the incidence but if the *P. gingivalis* story is correct the recent reduction in community dentistry and the gradual phasing out of NHS dental care by squeezing the income of dental surgeons will have really dire results.

Worldwide as the population ages the incidence of Alzheimers increases. The population of the developed countries is around 1.3 billion. Perhaps the population of China can be added to that making a total of 2.7 billion people who are likely to reach the age at which Alzheimer's disease becomes a significant factor. If 1 in 8 of these develop Alzheimer's that results in over 4 million people dying from the condition each year. Assuming the *Porphyromonas gingivalis* story is correct the bug has probably overtaken the other infections as the primary infective cause of demise. If you add in the heart disease, stroke and diabetes it is almost certainly the present number one in the Western world whilst malaria rules supreme elsewhere.

References

1. We may finally know what causes Alzheimer's – and how to stop it https://www.newscientist.com/article/2191814-we-may-finally-know-what-causes-alzheimers-and-how-to-stop-it/   By Debora Mackenzie
2. https://www.devonlive.com/news/devon-news/bse-crisis-john-selywn-gummer-2122969
3. https://en.wikipedia.org/wiki/2013_horse_meat_scandal
4. Kuru https://medlineplus.gov/ency/article/001379.htm
5. https://en.wikipedia.org/wiki/Bovine_spongiform_encephalopathy#Epidemiology
6. Porphyromonas gingivalis in Alzheimer's disease brains: Evidence for disease causation and treatment with small-molecule inhibitors. Stephen S. Dominy et al https://advances.sciencemag.org/content/5/1/eaau3333
7. The Eucharist (Service of holy communion) Book of Common Prayer, Church of England.

Chapter 11

The Origin of the COVID-19 Virus (SARS-2 CoV)

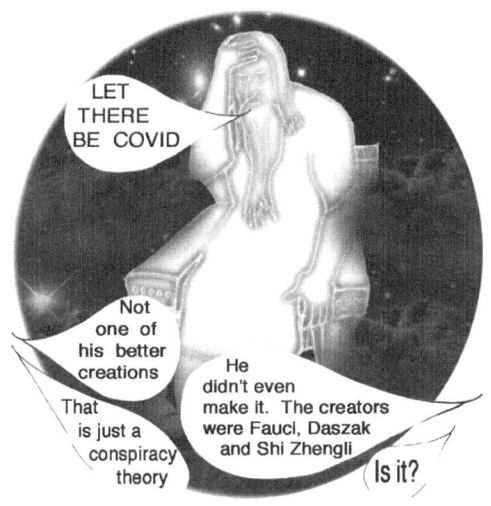

The Myth

In the beginning was the bat and the bat was with virus and the virus was with bat. Then came the pangolin and caught the virus from the bat. The pangolin was illegally plucked from its Eden and transported hundreds of miles to the Wuhan meat market and sold as an exotic food. Thus were sewn the seeds of the great pandemic of 2019 as the fallen human beings then passed the virus amongst themselves.

Facts and Likelihoods

The natural origin myth was foisted on us by the Chinese at the very beginning of the pandemic in January 2020. Initially I believed it but now, just as I stated in the first edition of this book (PANDEMIC, Clinical Press, June 2020) I totally reject the myth.

The pandemic has been sweeping round the world ever since December of 2019. In the first edition of this book I stated at the beginning of the chapter on COVID-19 : *"The pandemic is still in progress around the world as I write this chapter so the story will undoubtedly be changed. This is, however, firsthand experience as the sirens wail outside, the world is in lockdown and the mass graves are being filled as quickly as they are dug."* I did not suspect that more than a year later in 2021 the sentence would still be true. In the UK the vaccines have reduced the daily death toll to single figures but in the rest of the world the sirens wail and the mass graves are still being filled. So how did it really start? What was the origin of the SARS-2 COVID-19 virus? Here is by far the most likely version of events based on the huge body of information I have read.

Bats harbour many viruses including many species of coronavirus. A team from Wuhan were studying coronaviruses because of the Severe Acute Respiratory Syndrome (SARS-CoV-1) outbreak in 2003 in Yunnan province, China and the Middle East Respiratory Syndrome (MERS) of 2012 in Saudi Arabia. The team

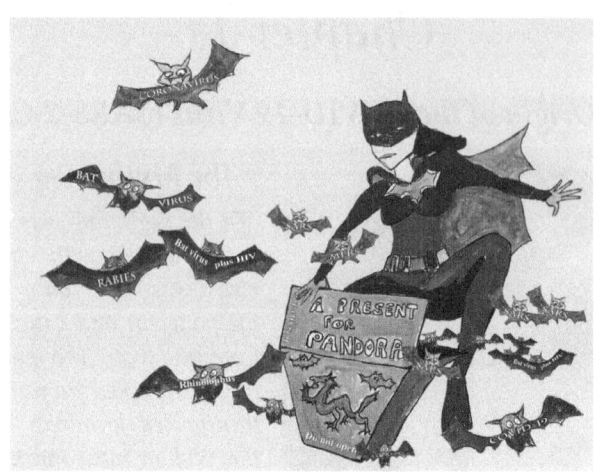

collected over two hundred different species of coronavirus but they were not particularly infective to human beings.

In 2014 the Wuhan-based virologist Shi Zhengli (known as the Bat Woman) and her team were offered large sums of money to perform Gain of Function (GoF) studies on the viruses. Making the viruses infective between humanised mice was the aim. Essentially they were making another disease (MAD) and this is the acronym I believe that kind of work deserves.

Dr. Peter Daszak, President of EcoHealth Alliance, a US-based organisation that conducts research and outreach programs on global health, had been provided with some of the money (about $600,000) by Dr Fauci, Director of the National Institute of Allergies and Infectious Diseases, part of the USA's NIH, because the research in the USA was stymied by a moratorium. Too many outbreaks of novel viruses had occurred from the US based virology laboratories so the Obama administration had called for a halt on the research in 2014. Over a million dollars had been given to EcoHealth Alliance by the US Agency for International Development (USAID) for a sub-agreement with the Wuhan Institute of Virology. Funding also came from the US Department of Defense. It is clear that the US State Department officials did not realise the threat that China represented.

China under Xi Jinping is a very different place compared with the liberalising leaders for the previous thirty years. Under Xi Jinping there have been far-ranging measures to enforce party discipline, crackdowns on dissent in Hong Kong, border skirmishes with India and major threats to the security of Taiwan.

Jinping is more like Mao Zedong than any leader since Mao died. In 2018 Jinping abolished the presidential term limits. Under his rule there has been a deterioration in human rights, increased censorship and mass surveillance.

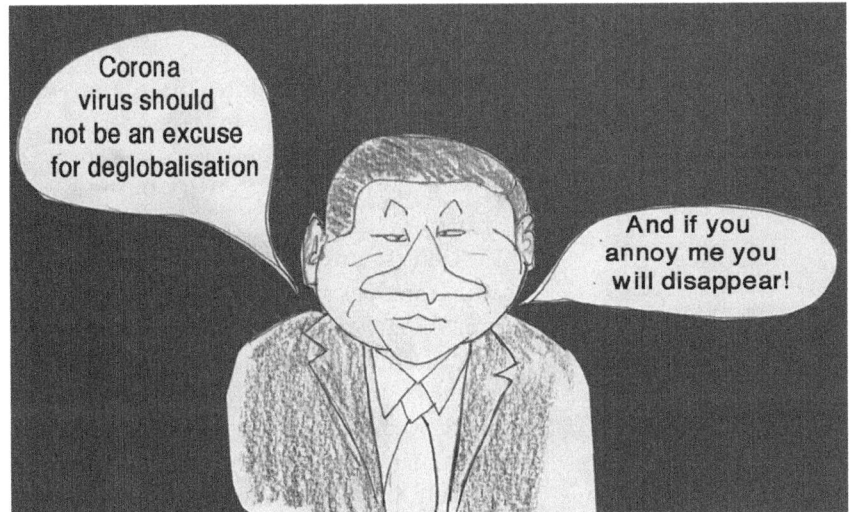

Xi Jinping assumed the office of president of China in 2013. In 2015 the Chinese military were looking at the possibility of weaponising a coronavirus. Subsequently they also had at least one laboratory in Wuhan experimenting with the viruses. A new building had been devised for virology research and the project was initially a joint venture between the Chinese and French. France provided the laboratory's design, biosafety training and most of its technology but when the building was completed in 2017 the French, much to their annoyance, were chucked out and, presumably, the Chinese military were moved in. The French politicians had backed the project but their security experts were against the project and were proven right. They had been warning the USA about the potential security risks from 2015 onwards.

Gain of Function (or MAD) studies were used to make the viruses infective between humanised mice on the assumption that if they could be so adapted it showed that they were potentially harmful to human beings. And the work was successful as reported by Daszak and Shi Zhengli in 2017 to 2019. In 2018, however, US officials who had visited the lab were told they would not be allowed to return and they therefore warned the US Government that there were major safety concerns.

In September 2019 some virologists in Wuhan had a peculiar respiratory infection. By October it was a growing and alarming problem and in December Dr Ai Fen, director of the emergency department at Wuhan Central hospital, was reprimanded after alerting her superiors and colleagues of a Sars-like virus seen in patients.

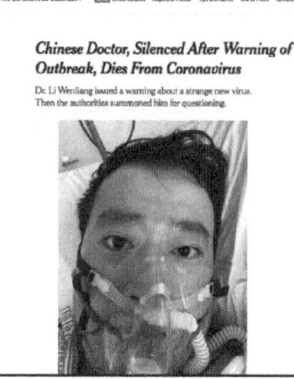

Dr Li Wenliang

Dr Li Wenliang, an ophthalmologist, was not party to these discussions between the hospital and government and warned friends on social media about the epidemic in December 2019. He was silenced by the authorities and officially was said to have died from COVID-19 on January 31st 2020.

The Chinese government allowed Chinese New Year celebrations to continue in Wuhan whilst quarantining the city and preventing its spread to the rest of China. They did, however, mysteriously allow people to fly out of Wuhan to the rest of the world. Very soon there were outbreaks of the new virus in many different cities around the world.

Eventually the WHO had to break ranks with the Chinese government and admit that the disease could spread between human beings and that it was reaching emergency proportions. China continued to tell the world that the virus could not be transmitted from person to person but eventually it was clear that it was easily transmitted that way, something that the Chinese had known from the start of the outbreak. China immediately stated that the virus had evolved naturally and that the intermediate host was the pangolin. In fact no pangolin has been shown to harbour the virus and the nail in the coffin of the natural evolution myth is the fact that bats cannot be infected with COVID-19.

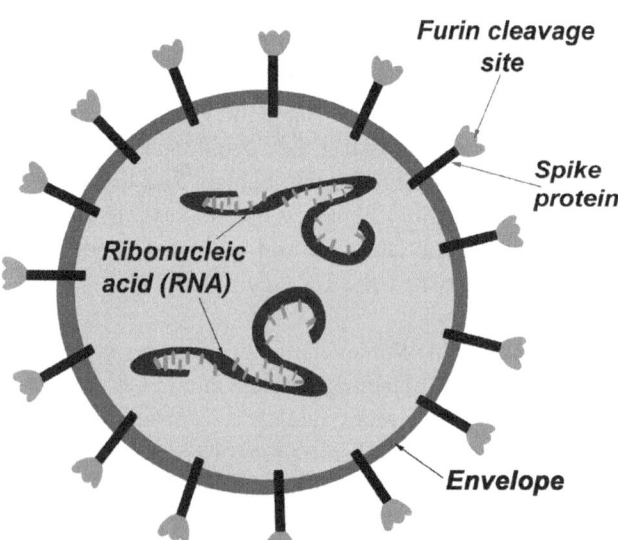

RNA is contained centrally in the virus. The spike glycoprotein has a potential cleavage site for furin proteases. This is essential for entry into the human cells. The nearest related bat virus does not have this site and SARS-CoV-2 cannot infect bat cells

The COVID-19 virus has a Furin cleavage site on the spike proteins. The virus attaches to the human Angiotensin Converting Enzyme 2 (ACE2) receptor. These receptors are part of the system that controls the blood pressure and are present in every blood vessel in the human body and also in many organs.

The Furin cleavage site helps the splitting of the spike which permits the RNA to enter the cell. The COVID-19 Furin cleavage site is unique to that coronavirus and is not present in any of the natural coronaviruses but similar sites are seen in other viruses pathogenic to human beings such as avian influenza, HIV and Ebola. The Chinese virologists reported success in adding similar spike proteins to other coronaviruses and making them infective in humanised mice which directly implies they were pathogenic to human beings. Daszak, in an interview, stated that adding the spike protein was easy.

In January 2020 virologist Kristian Andersen emailed Dr Fauci to tell him that there were some features of the virus that looked engineered and were "inconsistent with expectations from evolutionary theory". A flurry of emails and Zoom conferences between Fauci and colleagues then took place.

How Could A Virus Escape?

There are two theories as to how the virus escaped from the laboratories. The first is that the escape occurred because the virus was being cultivated and worked on using biosafety-level 2 at best and that the safety regime was extremely poor. This is backed up by the fact that a report by the funding US donors in 2018 had spotted the lax behaviour and reported back to President Trump to that effect.

The second possibility is strongly endorsed by Dr Scarlett Yan, the Hong Kong virologist who escaped to the USA. She makes a good case that the military virologists had already proven that the COVID-19 could infect humanised mice and that they were trying it out on prisoners when it escaped.

It is also interesting to note that Shi Zhengli and her team had tried to make a vaccine to combat the coronaviruses and had searched for drugs against them. Daszak reported that these efforts were unsuccessful but by midsummer of 2020 the Chinese were already immunising their airport staff. The Chinese vaccines are based on inactivated COVID-19.

Conspiracy Theory or Conspiracy?

By March 2020 Kristian Andersen published a paper in Nature Medicine stating, in a bewildering about turn, that it was highly unlikely that the COVID-19 virus had been made in a laboratory. He used as proof that his analysis showed that the virus was not perfectly adapted to infecting human beings which he believed it would be if it was made in a laboratory. The ability of the virus to infect all races and ages of people has proven that assertion to be completely incorrect.

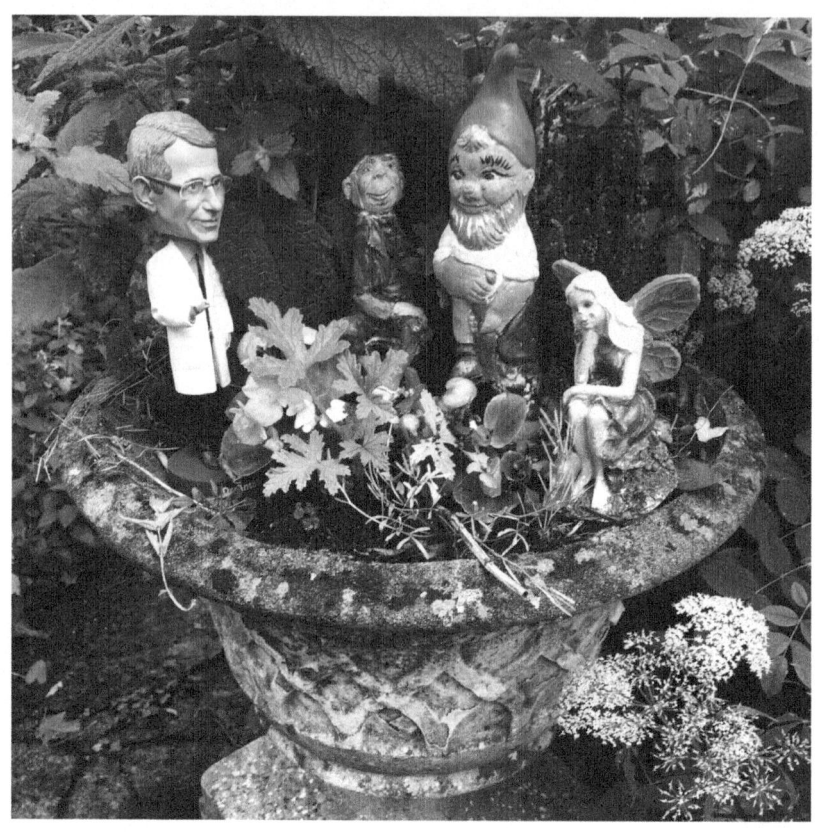

Dr Fauci meets the research team of Kristian Andersen.
From Left to Right: Dr Fauci. Larry the Leprechaun, Norman the Gnome and the Tooth Fairy. Fauci decides that they have done so well that they should be awarded a huge grant in order to set up a new Andersen Institute.

In April of 2020 Peter Daszak masterminded a letter in the Lancet casting people as conspiracy theorists if they thought that the virus may have arisen in the adjacent Wuhan laboratory, the only place in China that was studying the coronaviruses.

When I tell people about the laboratory escape theory of the origin of the virus I am frequently confronted with the accusation that this is just a conspiracy theory and obviously untrue. I have been accused of being naive for accepting such rubbish.

But why is the above section considered to be a conspiracy theory? Simply because the Lancet and Nature Medicine cast it as such and told people that

Table 1 Some examples of Escaped Laboratory Viruses

Date	Country	Virus	Outcome
1966	Birmingham UK	Smallpox	72 cases, no deaths
1971	Soviet Union	Smallpox	10 cases 3 fatal
1972	London UK	Smallpox	4 cases 2 deaths
1977	Russia and China	H1N1 Influenza	Pandemic which returned in 2009 as Swine Flu
1978	Birmingham UK	Smallpox	The last person to die from Smallpox
1995	Venezuela	Equine encephalitis	major equine epizootics and epidemic
2003-2017	China	SARS	six documented SARS disease outbreaks originating from research laboratories, including four in China. These outbreaks caused thirteen individual infections and one death
2007	Purbright UK	Foot and Mouth disease	Epidemic in British cattle
2015	USA	Anthrax	US Department of Defense accidentally shipped live anthrax spores to labs in nine US states and a US military base in South Korea

conspiracy theories are discriminatory and wrong. This has been reinforced via the media. I had to change my mind about the origin but many people find this is impossible to do, partly because Trump supported the theory. This is how I reported my conversion to "conspiracy theorist" on my Facebook pages:

April 24th 2020

So do I still believe the post I made in March that the virus was not engineered? That was based on a paper in Nature …..I now have sound reasons to doubt that paper. It is clear that the virologists at the Wuhan Virology Institute were studying bat viruses exceedingly similar, if not identical, to COVID-19. The first few cases had contact with the virology institute but not the meat market. More to follow:

All of the statements in this chapter about the development of coronaviruses using Gain of Function studies can be proven from the extensive scientific literature that Peter Daszak and Shi Zhengli have written on the subject and the interviews they have given…….except, of course, the paragraphs in which I state that the virus escaped. That this is the case is so highly likely that estimates of the probability using a super-computer and Bayesian statistics showed a greater than 99% chance that the lab leak is correct.

Daszak has gone out of his way to claim that the virus could not have possibly escaped from a laboratory on the spurious grounds that such escapes are so rare. Ever since virology started viruses have easily escaped from the labs. For example a report by Dr. George Packer in 1931 showed that thirty-two lab workers had been infected with Yellow Fever when examining it with four deaths.

It would be hoped that lessons had been learnt and that now such occurrences would be rare. That is not the case. The moratorium put on the research in 2014 shows that viruses commonly escape from laboratories in the USA and Table 1 confirms it.

The references for the table refer to the year in the first column and are found at the end of the chapter.

The Cover-Up

It was immediately apparent to the Chinese virologists that the virus was likely to have escaped from one of their laboratories. Shi, the Batwoman, is said to have checked as soon as she returned to her laboratory but reported that the records did not demonstrate a leak. This cannot be verified and perhaps the last free words she made were when she queried whether the virus had leaked from the laboratory. The other two Wuhan virology laboratories have not been so forthcoming with their stories but it is undoubtedly true that the virologists must have been very worried. We can no longer find out as they have almost all disappeared.

Kristian Andersen may have discovered the "insertions" but hid the evidence.

Entirely separately from Andersen, Professor Gus Dalgleish (St Georges Hospital, London) and Berger Sorensen (Norway) noticed that the research from China and the references in the Andersen paper in Nature Medicine all suggested that the Wuhan Virology Institute had been making pathogenic coronaviruses. Moreover the Furin cleavage on the spike proteins and the charge on them was abnormal. It had never been seen in a wild coronavirus. Dalgleish and Sorensen wrote a reply to Andersen's paper in Nature Medicine but that esteemed journal refused to publish the letter! Later their evidence was published in a paper about vaccines that has now been downloaded a quarter of a million times, thus becoming one of the most downloaded papers in history!

As discussed above Peter Daszak masterminded a letter to the Lancet, persuading colleagues to sign it, stating that the virus was a normally evolved pathogen and could not have come from the laboratory. Not surprisingly he forgot to declare a conflict of interest (in that he and the team he funded were busy manipulating the viruses in the very lab that the COVID-19 may have escaped from). Perhaps other people on the letter forgot to mention that they were funded by the NIH which had, in turn, funded similar research elsewhere?

No outside investigation was initially permitted, the Wuhan laboratories were sterilised and the biowarfare expert for China put in charge of them. Eventually, one year too late, the WHO investigating team were allowed into China. When the results of their investigation came out they expressly ruled out any possibility of a lab leak but thought it might have arrived on frozen food from abroad! I thought they were simply like the ostriches in my cartoon, unwilling and too scared to take their heads out of the sand and thus not seeing the obvious evidence in front of them.

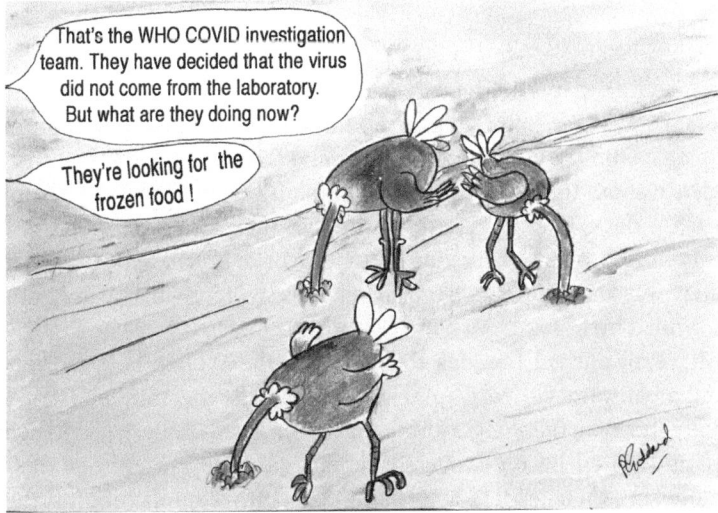

It was later revealed that the team was hand-picked by the Chinese and Daszak was a leading member. Again no mention was made of the conflict of interests. The team were told what to write by the Chinese authorities and they were not allowed to visit any of the sites in question, see any of the laboratory records, interview Chinese virologists and doctors or speak to any of the patients. So they were puppets.

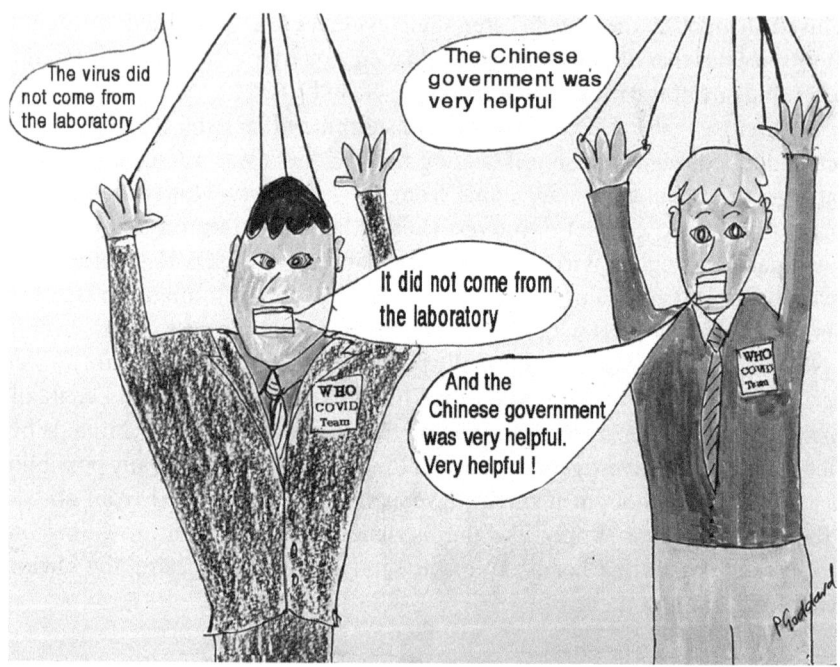

Thus it is clear that there have been several elements to the cover-up of the origin of the virus. The Chinese government covered up the original outbreak and Peter Daszak, with the Chinese authorities and the help of Shi Zhengli, obscured the evidence about the laboratory origin. Emails to and from Dr Anthony Fauci of the USA and Sir Jeremy Farrer show that they were also worried about a laboratory origin of the virus but chose to cover up this concern. Andersen knew there was an abnormal insertion but chose to accept a new institute (in his name!) funded by Fauci.

They have all pushed the idea that blaming the Wuhan laboratories is fake news and a conspiracy theory, implying that it must therefore be false. Twitter, Facebook and YouTube algorithms have removed material criticising the Chinese and this, I have discovered, is partly due to a multitude of Chinese lackeys obeying their leaders whim and constantly complaining on the social media, which in turn affects the algorithms that censor the material. In addition the billionaires who own the media are not blameless.

In fact the cover-up probably was a conspiracy and my comments therefore can be classed as a theory about a conspiracy, albeit a true one.

The fact that people disbelieve conspiracy theories does not mean that there are no conspiracies, it's just that most of them are cover-ups of cock-ups! The most famous conspiracy in recent history was Watergate and the main concern there was about the level of cover-up that was employed by the US government. Conspiracies exist because human beings do conspire together and the Chinese communist party are past masters at conspiracy!

Sinners or Saints? Geniuses or Donkeys?

Meanwhile the virologists continue to research using Gain of Function (GoF) studies. Fauci now claims these are not Gain of Function….he is trying to change the definition. As suggested earlier let us, instead, change the name. They are definitely Make Another Disease (MAD) studies carried out by MAD scientists.

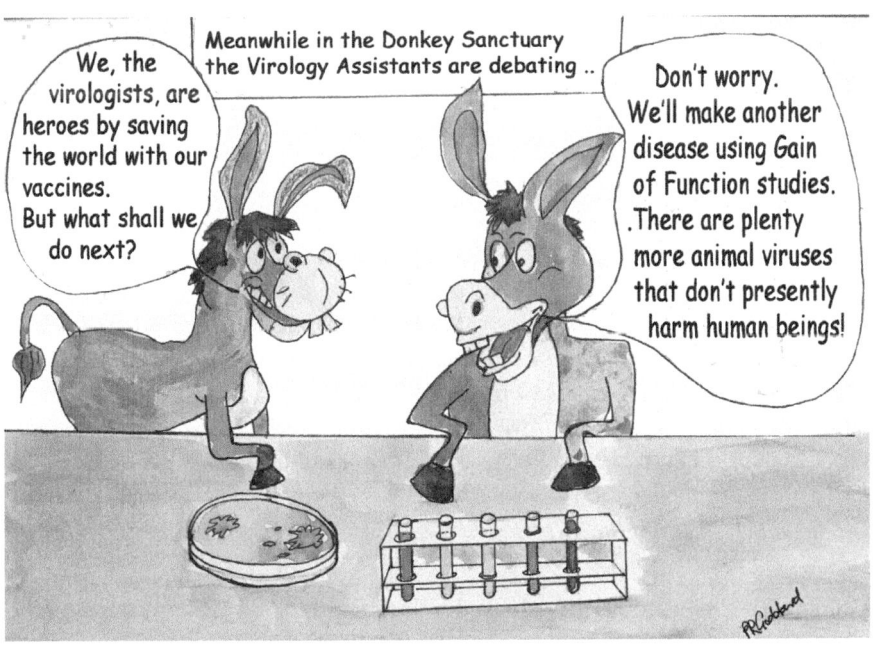

The Virologists in the Donkey Sanctuary continue with their Make Another Disease (MAD) research

The Conclusion Regarding the Origin of COVID-19
(as published in the first edition of PANDEMIC (June 2020))

The origin of SARS, MERs and SARS 2 (COVID-19)

You may recall there is a cartoon of Batwoman releasing bats and each bat has a virus name ascribed to it. Coronaviruses are a large family of viruses that normally affect mammals and birds. Many can be found in bats. Coronaviruses cause about a third of the common colds that human beings suffer from with the remaining two-thirds mostly due to rhinoviruses.

When I was a schoolboy I was most impressed by the science section in my comics, the Eagle, and Look and Learn, referring to research at Porton Down, ostensibly to find a cure for the common cold. In fact the psychopathic scientists at Porton Down were actually experimenting on volunteers and servicemen, telling them that they were looking for a cure but trying out nerve gas, mustard gas and other poisonous chemicals without informed consent.

So is there a cure for the common cold and are other coronaviruses dangerous?

No, there is presently no effective cure or safe vaccine and yes, they can be dangerous. Severe Acute Respiratory Syndrome (SARS), now known as SARS-CoV-1, came from bats in Yunnan province, China, and caused an outbreak between 2002-2004. It infected over eight thousand people killing 11% and is relatively closely related to SARS-2 COVID-19 coronavirus.

Middle Eastern respiratory syndrome (MERS) is due to another coronavirus and was first identified in Saudi Arabia in 2012. 35% of those affected died.

It was because of these outbreaks that I warned about novel coronaviruses in my Long Fox lecture in 2017. Coronaviruses were being manipulated by the Wuhan virologists and abnormal insertions made COVID-19 more infective in human beings. Apparently the Chinese Communist Party did not want the world to know what was going on so they destroyed any evidence regarding the true origin of the virus. Now it is alleged that they are trying to prevent discussion about the virus and are causing algorithms on social media to censor any mention of Wuhan and China's involvement in the inception of the pandemic.

Since that time vaccines have been developed and they will be the subject of Chapter 15. Whether or not they are safe is debatable.

Some of the famous people who died from COVID-19

- Dr. Dr Li Wenliang, 33, Wuhan ophthalmologist February 2020
- Dr. Alfa Sa'adu 68 London consultant physician and Nigerian chief, died March 2020
- Bobby Ball - comedian, 76, died October 28, 2020
- Eddie Large - comedian, 78, died April 2, 2020
- Captain Sir Tom Moore - British Army officer and charity fundraiser, 100, died February 2, 2021
- Alexander Thynn - 7th Marquess of Bath, 87, died April 4, 2020
- Dave Egerton - rugby player and coach,(Bath and England) 59, died February 8, 2021
- Dave Greenfield - musician, (Keyboards the Stranglers) 71, died May 3, 2020
- Norman Hunter - footballer (Bristol City, Leeds and England World Cup squad), 76, died April 17, 2020
- Tim Brooke-Taylor - actor and comedian, 79, died April 12, 2020
- Ty - rapper, 47, died May 7, 2020
- Roy Horn - magician and entertainer, 75, died May 8, 2020
- Alber Elbaz, 59, - Fashion designer. Died from complications of COVID-19 in Paris on April 24.
- Fred The Godson,41, The Bronx-born rapper died on 23 April
- Terrence McNally, award-winning playwright 24 March, aged 81
- Adam Schlesinger, 52, songwriter and co-frontman of US band Fountains of Wayne, on 1 April 2020
- Alan Merrill, 69 I Love Rock 'n' Roll songwriter

Further reading and references

1. https://www.nature.com/articles/d41586-020-00364-2
2. https://www.theguardian.com/commentisfree/2021/feb/22/i-was-on-the-whos-covid-mission-to-china-heres-what-we-found
3. https://doi.org/10.1016/S0140-6736(20)30418-9. | VOLUME 395, ISSUE 10226, E42-E43, MARCH 07, 2020 Statement in support of the scientists, public health professionals, and medical professionals of China combatting COVID-19. Charles Calisher, Dennis Carroll, Rita Colwell, Ronald B Corley, Peter Daszak, Christian Drosten et al.
4. https://www.youtube.com/watch?v=hAeX8v5a-Tc
5. https://www.thesun.co.uk/news/14499887/who-chief-covid-report-wuhan-lab-leak/
6. Andersen, K.G., Rambaut, A., Lipkin, W.I. et al. The proximal origin of SARS-CoV-2.Nat
7. Vineet D Menachery, Boyd L Yount Jr, Kari Debbink, Sudhakar Agnihothram, Lisa E Gralinski, Jessica A Plante, Rachel L Graham, Trevor Scobey, Xing-Yi Ge, Eric F Donaldson, Scott H Randell, Antonio Lanzavecchia, Wayne A Marasco, Zhengli-Li Shi & Ralph S Baric A SARS-like cluster of circulating bat coronaviruses shows potential for human emergence. Nat Med 21, 1508–1513 (2015). https://doi.org/10.1038/nm.398
8. Yan,Li-Meng.https://zenodo.org/record/4650821#.YGYXe9Xwa8W
9. Life on Mars? Chandra Wickramasinghe Clinical Press, Bristol 1997
10. Ren W et.al. (2007) [JOURNAL OF VIROLOGY, Feb. 2008, p. 1899–1907 Vol. 82, No. 4 doi:10.1128/JVI.01085-07]
11. Herfst, S. et al., 2012. Airborne transmission of influenza A/H5N1 virus between ferrets. Science, 22, pp. 1534-1541.
12. https://osp.od.nih.gov/wp-content/uploads/2016/02/Gain-of-Function%20Research%20Ethical%20Analysis%20White%20Paper%20by%20Michael%20Selgelid_0.pdf
13. https://logicandfacts.com/fauci-did-support-and-fund-creating-potential-bioweapons-in-china/
14. https://www.ecohealthalliance.org/personnel/dr-peter-daszak
15. https://www.sciencemag.org/sites/default/files/Shi%20Zhengli%20Q%26A.pdf
16. https://www.who.int/health-topics/severe-acute-respiratory-syndrome#tab=tab_1
17. https://en.wikipedia.org/wiki/Severe_acute_respiratory_syndrome
18. (https://en.wikipedia.org/wiki/Middle_East_respiratory_syndrome
19. (https://www.frontiersin.org/articles/10.3389/fpubh.2020.581569/full)
20. Wu F, Zhao S, Yu B, et al. A new coronavirus associated with human respiratory disease in China. Nature. 2020 Mar;579(7798):265-269. DOI: 10.1038/s41586-020-2008-3.
21. Zhou P, Yang XL, Wang XG, et al. A pneumonia outbreak associated with a new coronavirus of probable bat origin. Nature. 2020 Mar;579(7798):270-273. DOI:

10.1038/s41586-020-2012-7.
22. https://coronavirusexplained.ukri.org/en/article/cad0006/.
23. Hu B et al Discovery of a rich gene pool of bat SARS-related coronaviruses.https://journals.plos.org/plospathogens/article?id=10.1371/journal.ppat.1006698
24. https://metro.co.uk/2020/04/18/coronavirus-may-started-september-scientists-say-12576961/
25. https://www.dailymail.co.uk/news/article-8416163/Satellite-photos-hospital-car-park-China-suggests-pandemic-taking-hold-October.html
26. https://www.wsj.com/articles/chinas-bats-expert-says-her-wuhan-lab-wasnt-source-of-new-coronavirus-11587463204
27. https://www.kff.org/news-summary/cnn-reports-on-leaked-chinese-documents-showing-inconsistencies-in-pandemics-early-days-tedros-tells-nations-to-not-politicize-hunt-for-coronavirus-origins/
28. https://en.wikipedia.org/wiki/Li_Wenliang
29. https://www.hrw.org/news/2021/03/04/chinas-dangerous-game-around-COVID-19-vaccines
30. Sørensen B, Susrud A, Dalgleish AG (2020). Biovacc-19: A Candidate Vaccine for COVID-19 (SARS-CoV-2) Developed from Analysis of its General Method of Action for Infectivity. QRB Discovery, 1: e6, 1–11 https://doi.org/10.1017/qrd.2020.8
31. https://www.independentsciencenews.org/health/the-case-is-building-that-COVID-19-had-a-lab-origin/
32. (https://www.dailymail.co.uk/home/moslive/article-1184455/Battle-killer-bugs-The-lab-viruses-arent-just-welcome--theyre-breeding-them.html
33. tps://www.express.co.uk/news/world/1415703/Coronavirus-lab-leak-theory-bat-COVID-19-CDC-Wuhan-origin-latest-news-vn

References for the Table of Escaped Lab Viruses

1. 1966,1972,1977,1978.https://nationalpost.com/news/a-brief-terrifying-history-of-viruses-escaping-from-labs-70s-chinese-pandemic-was-a-lab-mistake
2. Ref 1971.https://en.wikipedia.org/wiki/1971_Aral_smallpox_incident
3. 1977,2009,1978, 1995, 2003 to 2017, 2015. https://www.independentsciencenews.org/health/the-case-is-building-that-COVID-19-had-a-lab-origin/2007. https://www.dailymail.co.uk/home/moslive/article-1184455/Battle-killer-bugs-The-lab-viruses-arent-just-welcome--theyre-breeding-them.html

References regarding Famous People

1. https://www.bristolpost.co.uk/news/celebs-tv/12-celebrity-coronavirus-victims-famous-5329505
2. https://news.sky.com/story/coronavirus-stars-and-notable-figures-who-have-died-after-contracting-COVID-19-11969431

Chapter 12
The COVID-19 Pandemic

The deaths from the COVID-19 pandemic rose very rapidly with the first wave peaking in the UK in April 2020. As the weather improved and the Spring turned into Summer the cases in the UK and across Europe plummeted.

Patients continued to suffer from the effects of COVID-19 after the initial infection has passed. This is known as Long Covid but includes "ongoing symptomatic COVID-19" (4 to 12 weeks after infection) and "post-COVID-19 syndrome" (more than 12 weeks after infection). See more about this later in the chapter.[1]

A table of symptoms and signs was published in the first edition in June 2020 and very little needs to be added or removed from it. It has been pointed out to me that the Chest CT findings do not just occur in the bases. That is absolutely the case....the classical appearances are lower zone peripheral opacities, often with a ground-glass appearance. However, as the disease progresses the opacification becomes more widespread so that severely ill patients rarely show the classical appearances.

Symptoms and signs of COVID-19
(First published in PANDEMIC first edition June 2020)
Resumé of the Clinical features of COVID-19 Coronavirus

When in January 2020 the WHO announced to the world that the novel coronavirus infection could be transmitted person to person we were told that it was a respiratory infection. The symptoms to look out for were dry cough and high fever.

But the virus can attack a large number of different areas in the human body. Many other signs, symptoms and complaints have been added to that list.

Adults
General
- Fever, Tiredness, Lethargy, Loss of appetite, Loss of weight.

Chest
- Continuous non-productive dry cough
- Less commonly productive cough
- Shortness of breath and difficulty in breathing
- Silent anoxia: pulse oximeter may show low oxygen levels.
- Chest CT shows areas of ground-glass opacification, mainly at the bases

Gut
- Diarrhoea
- Gastritis (inflammation of the stomach lining)

Skin
- Erythematous rash (red skin colouration)
- Chilblain-like appearances of the toes
- Horizontal ridging of the nails (a classical sign of severe trauma/illness)

Central Nervous System
- Loss of taste, loss of smell
- Numbness or tingling in the hands or feet, Venous thrombosis.
- Brain Fogging, Hallucinations, Transient Ischaemic Attack, Stroke
- Ascending paralysis (Guillain-Barré syndrome)

Heart and Vascular system
- Myocarditis: irregular pulse, tachycardia (fast pulse), chest pain, heart failure
- Vasculitis (blood vessel inflammation) and Disseminated Intravascular Coagulation (widespread clotting using up the clotting factors and leading to bleeding).

Liver
- Liver function abnormalities: Hepatitis. Liver failure

Renal:
- Kidney stones, Renal failure

Motor System
- Weakness of voluntary muscles and pain

Post-infection
- Numerous symptoms including Chronic fatigue syndrome, gastro-intestinal symptoms, lingering bacterial/fungal infections, finger and toenail symptoms. Oral problems.

Childhood:
- Usually mild cold-like symptoms of runny nose and cough
- Occasionally Kawasaki-like syndrome: Paediatric Inflammatory Multisystem Syndrome with vasculitis of small vessels.

****

The Waves of the Pandemic

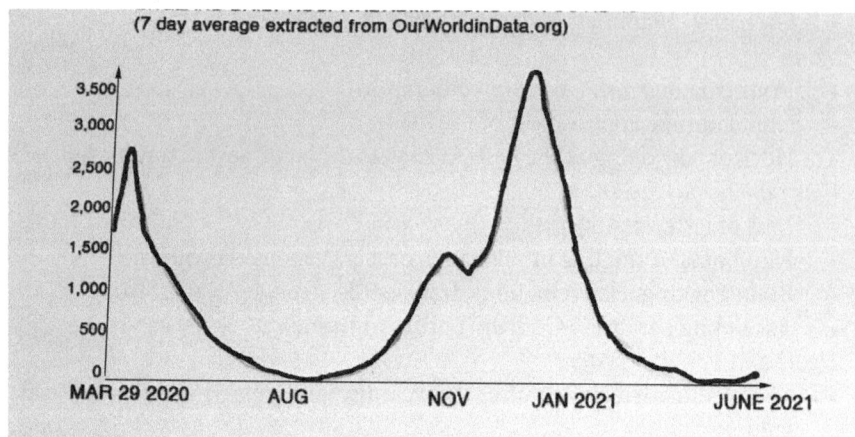

England : Daily Hospital Admissions for COVID-19

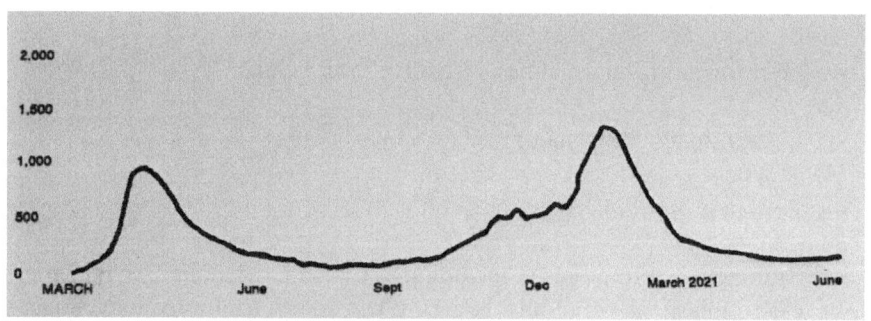

Chart of Deaths UK

When I wrote the first edition the first wave of the pandemic in the UK had ended. Approximately 60,000 people had died in the UK, about one in a thousand of the population and at that point I predicted that there would be a second wave starting in October but I did not think it would be as deadly as the first.

My prediction was initially correct. A second wave appeared, peaked at the end of November at a lower peak than in April and started to fall at the beginning of December. Then a strange thing happened...the cases started to surge again and reached a peak towards the end of January before dropping very quickly as the vaccines began to work.

As I write there are still cases sporadically appearing all over the UK but in considerably fewer numbers than before and daily deaths, which peaked at a rolling average of just over eighteen hundred in January, are now down in double or even as low as single figures per day.

Analysis of the charts displayed here shows that the December surge is in fact a third wave. The reason for the upswing in cases was a new variant known colloquially as the Kent variant. The official names for the Kent variant is B.1.1.7 but it is also known as VOC ("variant of concern") 202012/01 or as the Alpha variant.

The Kent variant is 70% more transmissible than the original COVID-19 and is also deadlier. [2] The greater ability to infect people seems to be due to more vigorous virus replication in the nasal passages leading to violent sneezing that spreads the virus far and wide. The Kent variant has spread to Europe creating a third wave in many of the European countries.

To recap: the Kent variant (Alpha) causes paroxysmal sneezing in the early stages whereas a runny nose was a feature in children with the original COVID-19 and not a particular concern in adults. Runny nose is also a feature with the Indian variant (Delta).

To date (August 7th 2021) around 130,000 people have died from COVID-19 in the UK, just over 1 in 500 of the population.

The first chart shows the daily hospital admissions for England and the second chart the seven day running average of deaths in the UK from the COVID-19 pandemic (people dying within 28 days of a positive test).

Let us go over this again: there is considerable argument over the definition of deaths from COVID-19 since any death, even from an accident, within the 28 days after testing positive may be counted as a Covid death. However the importance of the charts lies not in the actual figures but in the shape of the curves. Whilst the UK government wittered on about avoiding a third wave, as mentioned earlier we were already in the third wave and it was due to the Kent variant. Now we are in the fourth wave which has been due to the Indian or Delta variant. If the charts are examined a slight upsurge of admissions and deaths is noticeable in June and this has continued. The number of admissions to hospital rose to a low peak in July and started to fall in August. Deaths obviously lag behind admissions and they peaked in the first week of August 2021.

Variants had appeared in Brazil, South Africa and India. In the UK the upswing in cases due to the Delta variant translated into only a small upswing in deaths and this has been attributed to the vaccination programme. The majority of the hospital admissions are people who have not been vaccinated.

Interestingly the South African Beta variant appears to have been ousted in the UK by the Delta variant.

Around 560,000 Brazilians have now died from COVID-19—13% of the world's COVID-19 deaths [3] and more than the country's entire AIDS epidemic. With a population of 214 million about 1 in 380 have died and that is somewhat worse than the UK. This is probably due to their slower uptake of vaccination. The Chileans, most unfortunately, are suffering from a major epidemic of the Lambda variant which was first detected in Peru. This appears to be resistant to the immune response engendered by the Chinese vaccines which had been administered very efficiently in Chile. There is more about this in the section on vaccines.

We will see further waves in the UK due to new variants but hopefully they will be reduced by the vaccines and by the judicious use of repurposed drugs and supplements such as Vitamin D3.

Analysis of Excess Deaths in England March to July 2020

Excess Deaths in 3 areas of England 20 March 2020 to 31 July 2020

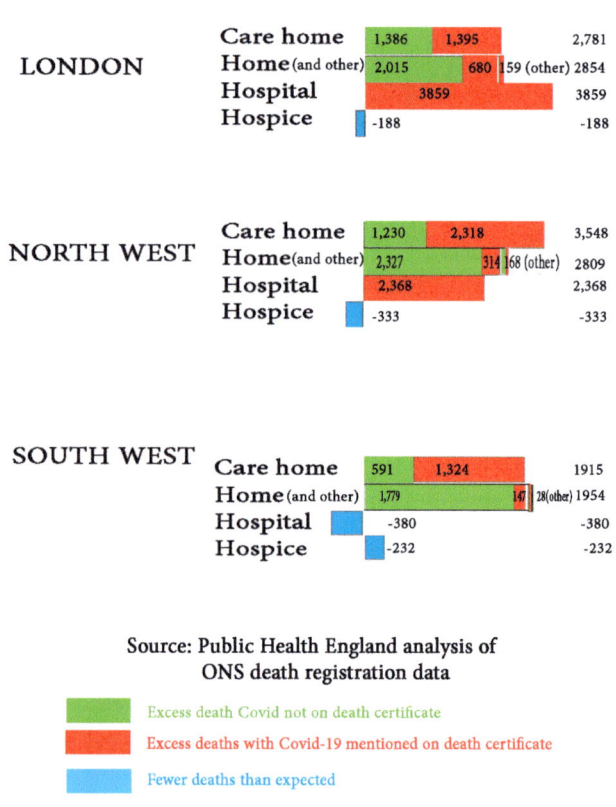

Source: Public Health England analysis of ONS death registration data

- Excess death Covid not on death certificate
- Excess deaths with Covid-19 mentioned on death certificate
- Fewer deaths than expected

The number of admissions and deaths does not tell the whole story. It is important to consider the excess deaths compared with the average for the time of year. Three areas are compared in the chart for the first lockdown period, March to July 2020.

Analysing the statistics [4] of excess deaths in the UK during the previous lockdown of March to July, in particular focussing on three areas, London, the North West and the South West illuminates what happened during the first wave of the COVID-19 pandemic in the UK..

A large number of cases of deaths from COVID-19 were being reported in London, somewhat fewer in the North West and far fewer in the South West. The excess death statistics bear this out with around 6000 excess deaths attributed to COVID-19 in London, 5,000 in North West and only 1500 in the South West. The populations are 9.3 million, 7.3 million and 5.6 million respectively. Correcting this per million puts the North West on top at 684, London next at 645 but the South West way behind at 268 per million - less than half the number of cases.

Looking at the place of death is interesting. There are four main places: home, care homes, hospice and hospital.

In all three districts there were fewer deaths than usual in the hospices.

In London most excess deaths occurred in hospital and were due entirely to covid. Half the excess deaths in care homes were covid related and a third of those at home were due to covid.

In the North West the majority of the excess deaths from any cause occurred in care homes and two thirds of these were covid related. The excess deaths in hospital were all covid related and were equal in number to the covid deaths in care homes. One eighth of the excess deaths at home were covid related.

In contrast in the South West nearly all the excess deaths were in care homes. 70% of the excess deaths in the care homes were due to covid. Only one thirteenth (1/13) of the excess deaths at home were covid related. The hospitals in the south west had considerably fewer deaths than normal.

What can we make of all this? It looks as if the London hospitals held on to a lot of the patients with COVID-19 but at the other extreme the South West hospitals got rid of them to the care homes (where many died from the covid) and actively discouraged admissions (hence excess deaths at home from non-covid related conditions).

This is all a matter of surmising from statistics but I think it shows that the management of the hospitals in the south west were over zealous in protecting the NHS with the obvious result that they under-treated the population of the south west.

The statistics are based on death certificates and they are notoriously inaccurate. It is possible that many of the deaths at home that were not diagnosed as COVID-19 related may have actually have been misdiagnosed and the covid missed. It does however suggest that assiduously emptying the hospitals does lead to excess morbidity and mortality in the community. This is to be expected and it is to be hoped that the NHS can learn from its mistakes and during any future pandemic hospitals will continue to treat conditions other than just coronavirus. Otherwise we will not have been clapping the ongoing efforts of the National Health Service Health but applauding the inception of solely a half-hearted National Pandemic Service.

Long Covid

Over a million people in the UK have self-reported Long Covid [5].

The definition of Long Covid is rather woolly and can refer to anyone who has continuing symptoms a few weeks after having the virus. The figure of a million is undoubtedly a major under-estimate.

It includes "ongoing symptomatic COVID-19" (4 to 12 weeks after infection) and "post-COVID-19 syndrome" (more than 12 weeks after infection). In addition some people include the patients who are post-ventilation …. their symptoms will include all the usual after effects of being on a ventilator in intensive care. The fourth group of people with Long Covid are those with organ damage caused by the virus.

Four overlapping forms of *Long Covid*

- Post-viral fatigue syndrome
- Ongoing ill-health
- Post-ventilation: muscle wasting
- Organ damage: lung scarring, myocardial infarction, myocarditis, cerebro-vascular accidents (stroke), renal and other organ failure due to the cytokine storm

Test and Trace, Testing and Variant Analysis

Good test and trace would seem to be imperative if a pandemic is to be brought under control. In Chapter 4 I have reproduced my cartoon of a 14th century tracing app but here is a cartoon about Test and Trace consultants. Apparently Test and Trace Consultants have been paid £1000 per day (or possibly more?). So I have drawn one of the consultants looking at their nest egg!

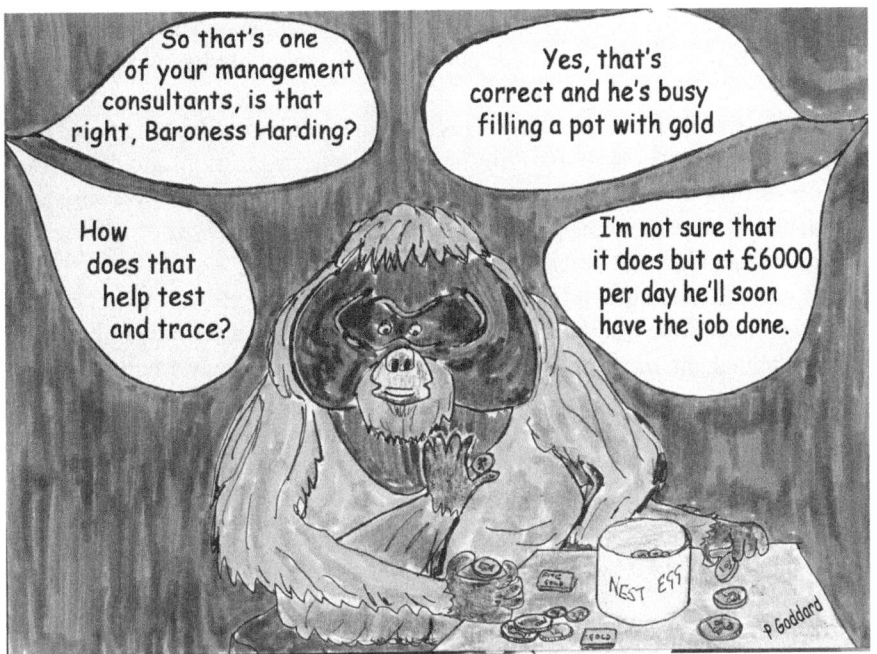

Unfortunately the track and trace that has been employed in the UK bore too much resemblance to the cartoon. Baroness Harding was put in charge of the UK Covid test and trace team and £37 billion has been spent on it. That is equivalent to three-quarters of the annual salary bill for the entire NHS yet the results have been dire.

There are people who are experts in test and trace. Medically the respiratory teams test for tuberculosis and trace contacts. The Sexually Transmitted Disease clinics do the same for STDs. The police try hard to trace criminals and have large computer systems to assist them in the task. So why was Baroness Harding, a novice in this field, entrusted with the task and why was it left up to commercial concerns? [6] As a BMJ blog points out the story could have been completely different. Volunteers would have been willing to run such a system, the vast expense avoided and the results much better. Here is their story: *"A small group of retired public health and primary care staff formed Sheffield Community Contact Tracers (SCCT) a year ago. We linked with a local community volunteer hub and the local Primary Care Network. We demonstrated in a small study that volunteers could be quickly and safely trained to undertake contact tracing of COVID-19 cases identified by local GPs. We ensured that cases and quarantined contacts were supported throughout their isolation."*

There is no convincing evidence that the enormous expense has done anything to halt the pandemic. If it had been successful we would not be onto the fourth wave.

However useless the test and trace has been in its attempt to halt the pandemic it is absolutely clear that it is ruining livelihoods, education and leisure of numerous people. Whole schools are being shut down by one positive case and the NHS app is even tracing people who live in the next door house but have not left their home!

As I write this paragraph the restrictions have been relaxed and have become voluntary but the test and trace continues and does not discriminate between the vaccinated and unvaccinated. NHS staff are, unsurprisingly, frequently near positive cases. So many are being told to self-isolate, each for ten days, that hospitals are dangerously under-staffed and personnel are removing the NHS app from their mobile phones. This is known as the Pingdemic because the NHS app goes *"ping"* to tell people that they must isolate for ten days because they have been near someone who has tested positive. Some supermarket shelves have emptied due to lack of delivery staff.

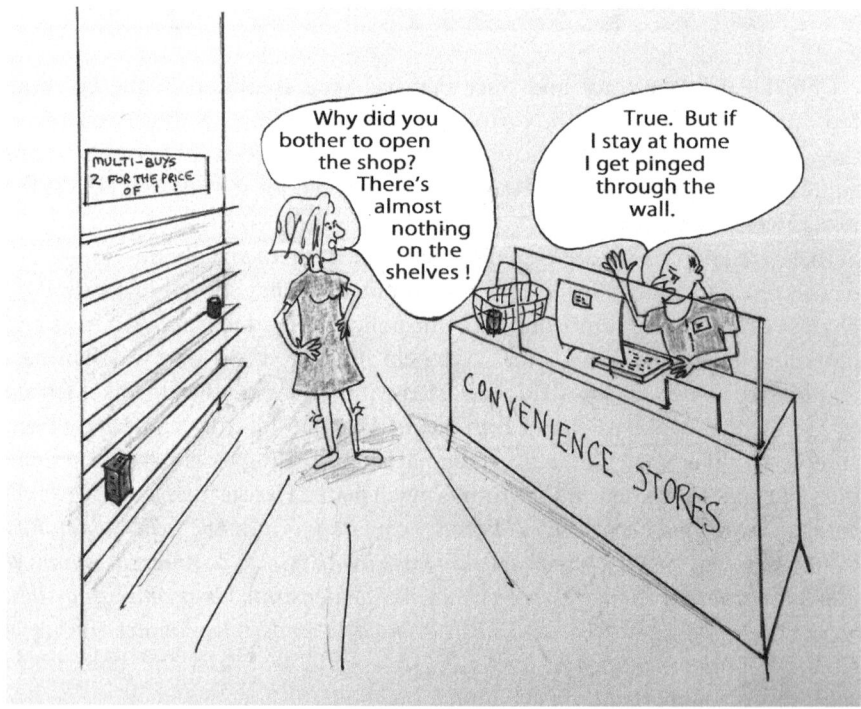

Variant analysis

Variant analysis, on the other hand, has been an unmitigated success. The UK has led the world in determining the presence and nature of the different variants.

Variants of Concern [6]
- Alpha B.1.1.7 and B.1.1.7 +E484K identified September 2020 The Kent variant which caused the third wave in the UK
- Beta B1.351 identified September 2020. South Africa
- Gamma R1 Brazil
- Delta B.1.617.2 India. The variant that is causing a fourth wave of cases in the UK but due to vaccines is not causing much hospitalisation as yet.

Variants of Interest
- Eta B.1.525 Nigeria. Identified December 2020
- Epsilon B.1.427/B.1.429 USA. Identified September 2020
- Theta P.3 The Philippines. Identified January 2021
- B.1.616 France
- Kappa B.1.617.1 India
- B.1.620 Unclear

And there are a whole lot more which are being monitored including the Peruvian Lambda variant (also known as C.37) which is sweeping through South America !

Why were the results in the UK so bad and why did so many people die?

The next chapter details the different responses to the pandemic around the world but here I will very briefly mention a few of the reasons that the death rate was so high in the UK. Later chapters will expand this answer but here is a brief resumé of the reasons:

- An unfit and unhealthy population. Low vitamin D levels, high incidence of obesity, high incidence of diabetes and many elderly people
- Refusal to let doctors use repurposed drugs
- Chronic underfunding of the NHS
- Discharge of sick patients into the nursing homes where there was initially no PPE, no testing and no medical support.
- Difficulty of seeing or even contacting general practitioners
- The initial lack of response by the Government and continuing mistakes (eg. they did not quarantine people from China at any time and in 2021 did not quarantine people arriving from India until thousands had arrived with the Delta variant.)

References

1. https://www.ons.gov.uk/peoplepopulationandcommunity/healthandsocialcare/conditionsanddiseases/bulletins/prevalenceofongoingsymptomsfollowingcoronaviruscovid19infectionintheuk/1april2021#-self-reported-long-covid
2. https://graphics.reuters.com/HEALTH-CORONAVIRUS/UK-VARIANT/ygdpzgblxvw/
3. https://www.bmj.com/content/373/bmj.n1227.
4. Public health England analysis of ONS death registration data
5. https://www.ons.gov.uk/peoplepopulationandcommunity/healthandsocialcare/conditionsanddiseases/bulletins/prevalenceofongoingsymptomsfollowingcoronaviruscovid19infectionintheuk/1april2021#-self-reported-long-covid
6. https://blogs.bmj.com/bmj/2021/03/19/COVID-19-test-and-trace-scandal-its-not-too-late-to-change-the-story/
7. https://www.ecdc.europa.eu/en/COVID-19/variants-concernHistorians Flavius

Chapter 13
The Responses to the COVID-19 Pandemic
Quarantine, Lockdown, Self-isolation, Social distancing, Shielding, Curfew, Test and Trace

When the COVID-19 pandemic was beginning many countries around the Pacific rim closed their borders to visitors. People returning from overseas were made to properly quarantine which involves being shut up in an enclosed space with no direct contact with anybody, not even the hotel staff / prison guards.

Quarantine: The term Quarantine is derived from the Venetian word "quarantena" meaning 'forty days'. This was the period for which people being quarantined would be placed in isolation. The term 'quarantine' came into use in England during the 17th century when the Plague was rife.

Did we quarantine people in the UK in 2020? No..... we asked people to self-isolate and brought in 'lockdowns'. So what do these terms mean?

Self-isolation is the situation when somebody deemed to either be a risk due to the possibility that they may be infectious (or perhaps are known to be having tested positive to a disease) isolates themselves from everybody except the very few people in their 'support group' or household. If they are known to be infected the people that they have been in contact may also be told to self-isolate. They must stay at home. In the UK self-isolation is a legal requirement if instigated by the NHS Test and Trace team or by the NHS COVID-19 app.

Social distancing: This was brought in to reduce spread of virus in the general population. The main techniques are the use of barriers, distance, time and cleanliness.
- Barriers: including masks, visors, gloves and screens.
- Distance: staying at least two metres away from people.
- Time: stay for as short a time as necessary in areas where there are crowds or potential risk (such as shops).
- Cleanliness: washing hands with soap and water is the most important process. Using hand gel or sanitiser if soap and water are not available.

Shielding is for people who are deemed to be at risk from infection. People who were considered as highly vulnerable were asked to work from home if possible and to avoid public transport during busy periods. They can use the same techniques as social distancing (barriers, distance, time and cleanliness). Voluntary social distancing, self-isolation and shielding were promoted to the public as a necessity from the middle of March 2020. It was deemed to be a failure and the statisticians predicted a vast increase in the number of deaths so on the 23rd of the same month Boris Johnson announced a lockdown and this became law on 26th March.

Lockdown: In the UK lockdowns businesses were closed, parks and play areas locked up and activities restricted. People were not allowed to meet with other households and the wearing of masks in public places was made mandatory. Quarantine may appear conceptually similar to lockdown but on examination it is actually the opposite. In lockdown the whole population of an area, such as a country or state, has their activity reduced but not completely stopped. In quarantine just those who are a risk to the population are constrained and prevented from leaving the place of confinement. The activity of those who are a contagion risk to the population is completely curtailed for a short determined period in quarantine compared with the activity of those who are at risk from a contagion being partially reduced for an often indeterminate period in lockdown.

Curfew refers to a time in the day when people must stay in at home or wherever they are residing. Curfews were not brought into action in the UK but was officially used in places such as Barbados.

Did the measures work?

The countries that instituted strict quarantine had very few cases of COVID-19. They are now vaccinating their population (rather too slowly) and will hopefully avoid a large death toll completely.

In the UK no quarantine was brought in until a year too late and even then it is very patchy with a government controlled "traffic light" scheme. Some countries (green) require no quarantine, some partial quarantine (amber) and some complete quarantine (red) in a hotel chosen by the government. But business people on essential trips can avoid quarantine as long as they have tested negative at least once on their trip. Moreover when we were travelling there was plenty of crossover and contact between people going to different places which must allow spread of disease.

Most people have still not been out of the UK for almost eighteen months whereas we have been to Germany, Spain and Barbados completely legally. This did involve testing and, in Barbados, quarantine in a designated hotel. Luckily we tested negative throughout. If we had tested positive we would have been taken in a military ambulance under guard to the detention centre in the north of the country until we had tested negative.

No such controls existed in the UK when we returned from Germany, Spain and Barbados although they may do now, eighteen months too late, depending

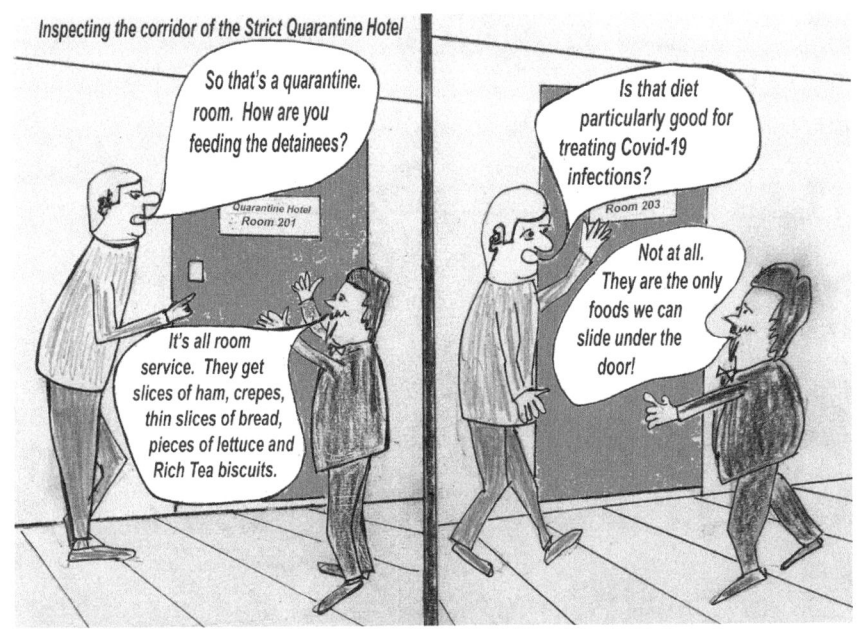

In the Corridors of the Quarantine Hotel

on which country you are flying from. People flying into the UK from the countries designated as a high infection risk (Red) have to stay in a Government designated quarantine hotel.

The UK regulations regarding quarantining are very peculiar. Some travellers do not have to quarantine because they are doing "essential work". One such employee I spoke to worked for a company leasing aircraft. Because he was officially an aircraft engineer his work was deemed as essential, he understood that he had to test negative once then could travel into any country and back to the UK without quarantining. This seems to apply to aircraft crew as well.

A Crown servant or government contractor travelling to the UK for essential government work in the UK or returning from conducting such work outside the UK can receive a letter from the Government and gain exemption from quarantining. They must, however, test negative on COVID-19 testing before travelling to the UK.[1]

These exemptions are considered necessary or air travel and international business could not continue. What a good job it is that the COVID-19 is able to read the small print and will not spread if you have the appropriate exemption letter!

Reference (1) www.gov.uk Jobs that qualify for travel exemptions

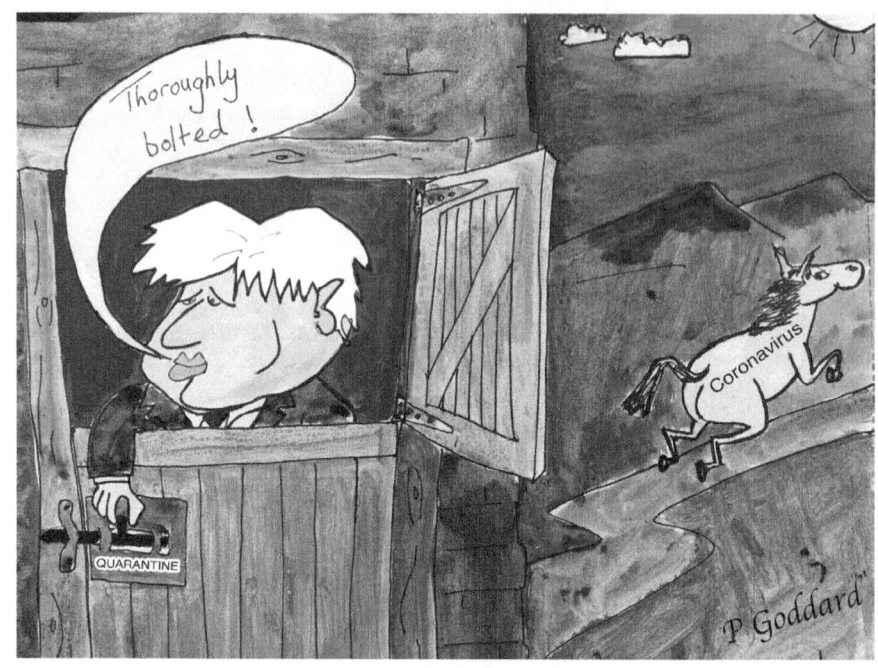

Boris has hemmed himself in, quarantining people over a year too late and making people isolate if "pinged" by the NHS test and trace app

I really don't think that officialdom understands the idea of quarantine. If a genuine and total quarantine had been brought into play at the beginning of the pandemic in late 2019 or early 2020 we may have saved 120,000 deaths (though arguably many of the actual victims would have died in 2020 anyway from other causes.) If the scientists who knew about the true origins of the virus had warned the governments they would have instituted quarantine on anybody from China. Quarantining travellers eighteen months after the virus has swept the country may keep out a few variants but it is the vaccination programme that does appear to have succeeded in overwhelmingly reducing the death rate even from the newer variants. Quarantine that includes government exemptions is not quarantine at all: it is just a way of punishing holiday travellers.

As I write this Boris is having to self-isolate despite having previously had COVID-19 and having been fully vaccinated. The horse had thoroughly bolted by the time he brought in quarantine and now he has been caught by his own self-isolation laws.

Absurd!

Was Lockdown effective and has Test and Trace made any useful contribution? What were the harmful effects on health and the economy from the first countrywide lockdowns in living memory? These questions will be answered in the next chapter

Masks

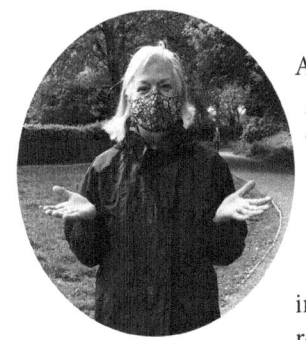

At the beginning of the pandemic we wore masks and gloves in public. Almost nobody else followed our example but at least they tended to shy away from us making the self-isolation quite effective. Wearing masks for more than a few minutes is bad for the health and there is very little evidence to support it. Despite this mask wearing in public enclosed spaces, including schools, became mandatory and has only recently been relaxed, though some public areas and transport still demand that a mask is worn.

Correctly worn mask

I have observed a lot of different methods of wearing a mandatory mask. Casually covering the chin or just the mouth is a common sight. Some jokers wear celebrity masks. I have not actually seen Dick Turpin but I can imagine the confusion.

I have seen a condom worn as shown but not recently!

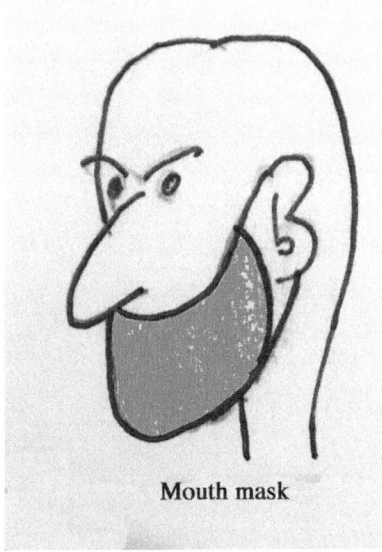

Mouth mask

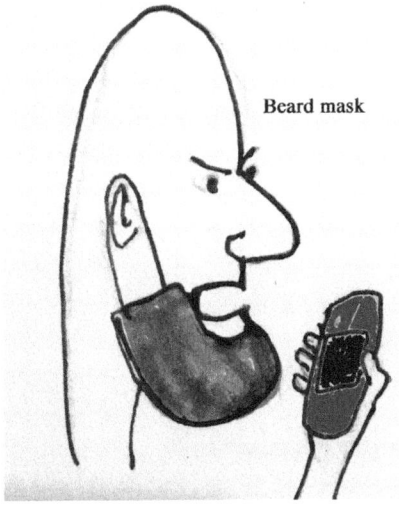

Beard mask

Celebrity Mask

Condom mask

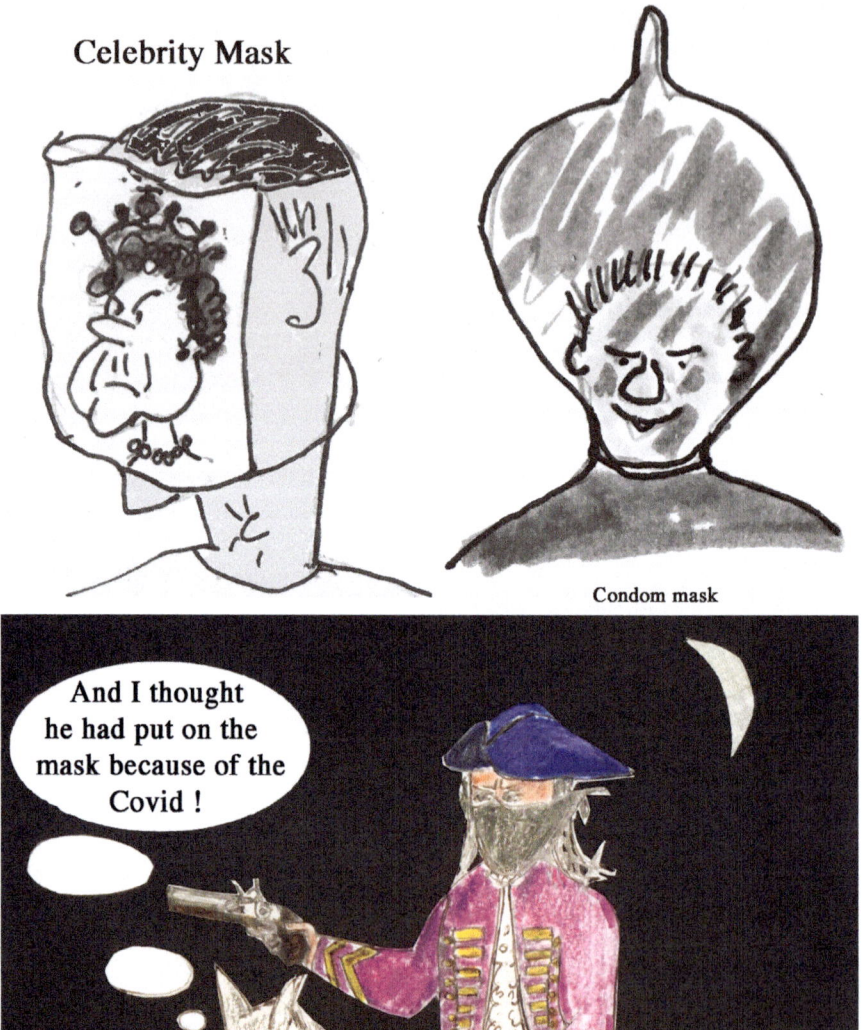

Dick Turpin confuses his horse

Chapter 14
The effects of lockdowns

The UK implemented the first lockdown in late March 2020. It lasted until June 2020. Most businesses were closed and employees put on a government backed furlough scheme.

In the following pages are a few of the pictures of lockdown, business premises closed and pavements and roads nearly deserted. More pictures were published in colour in the first edition of PANDEMIC.

LONDON UK

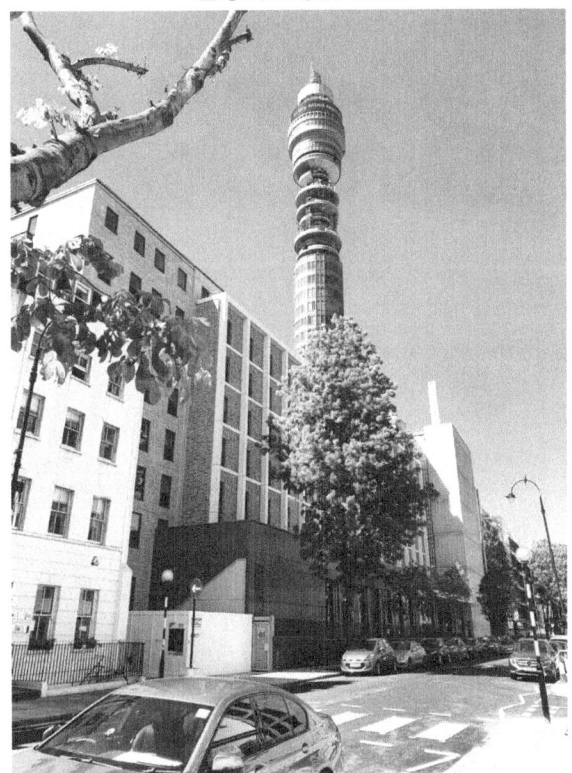

The Post Office Tower during Lockdown in London. No pedestrians, clear sky with no contrails and no clouds, and a message on the tower "Every mind matters".
Photograph © Mark Goddard 2020

BRISTOL UK

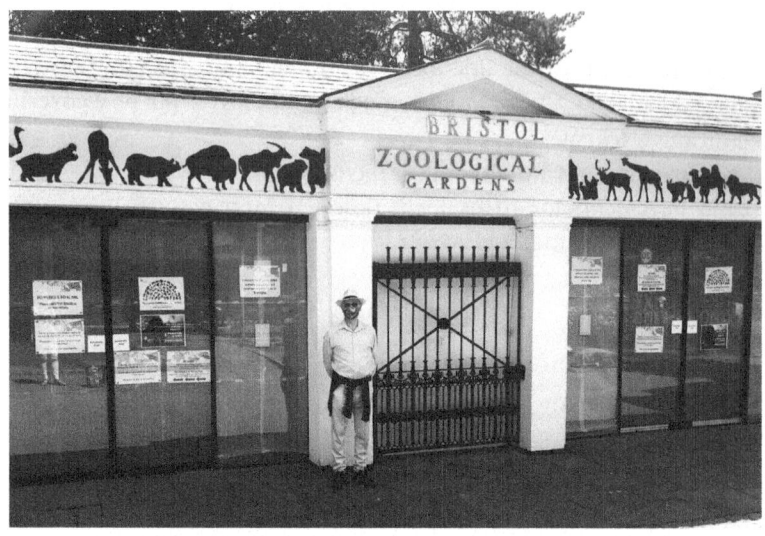

Bristol Zoo (founded 1835), closed during lockdowns. The zoo society announced in November 2020 that the Clifton site would close permanently at the end of 2022 and move to their other site at the Wild Place Project.

SCOTLAND UK

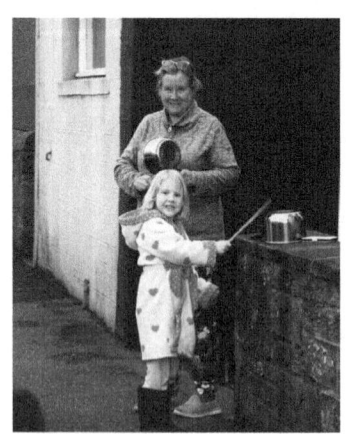

The NHS Clapping with Granny. The little girl's other grandmother had died from the COVID-19 infection and the clapping was good therapy.

© *photograph by Ian Crighton 2020*

ITALY

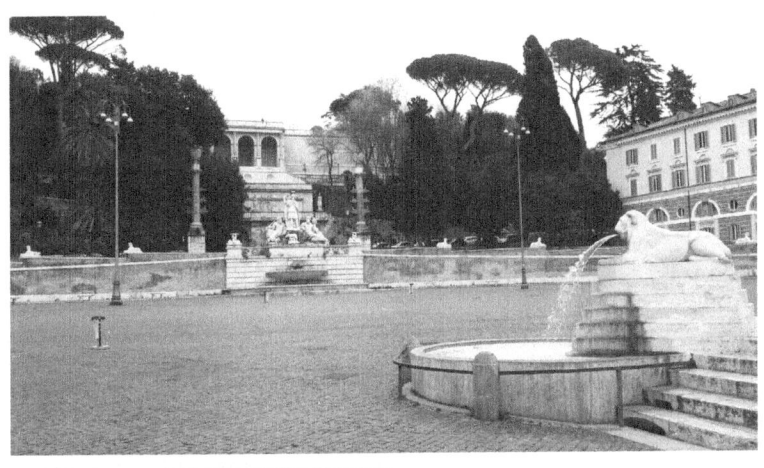

Above: Rome but nobody is roaming
© *Chris Holder 2020*

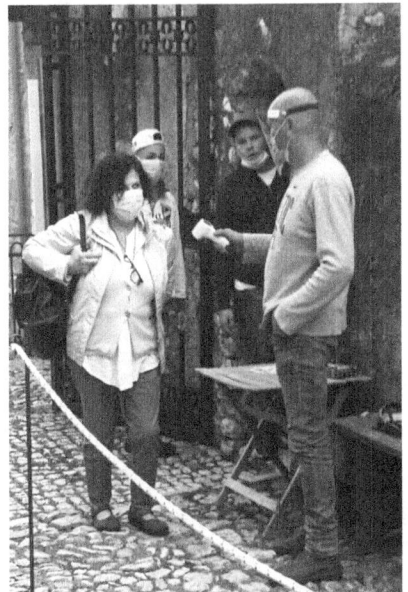

Left: Digital thermometer gun at Sermoneta Castle. Note the man with a "chin mask" : a common phenomenon !
© *Chris Holder 2020*

CHAMONIX, FRANCE

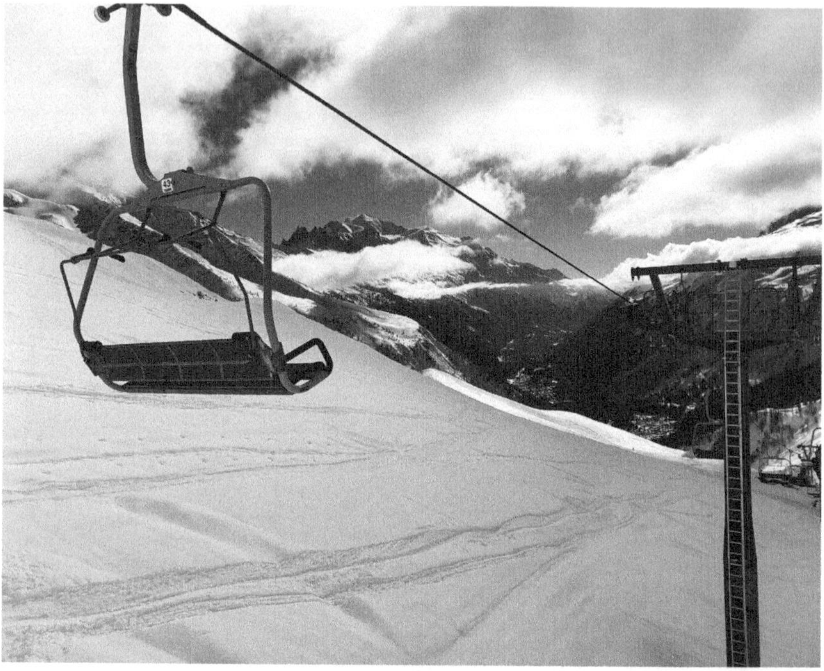

Above: Empty ski lifts and empty slopes

Right: On the 15th March in the small hours of the morning the French authorities closed the ski resorts. No hotels, no bars, no restaurants and no skiing. Many thousands of holidaymakers from the UK were flying in as the skiers were trying to leave. There was chaos at the airport!

Photographs
© Mark Goddard 2020

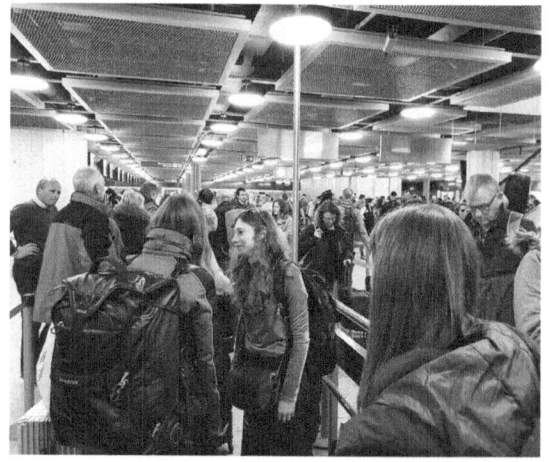

HOME SCHOOLING (GERMANY)

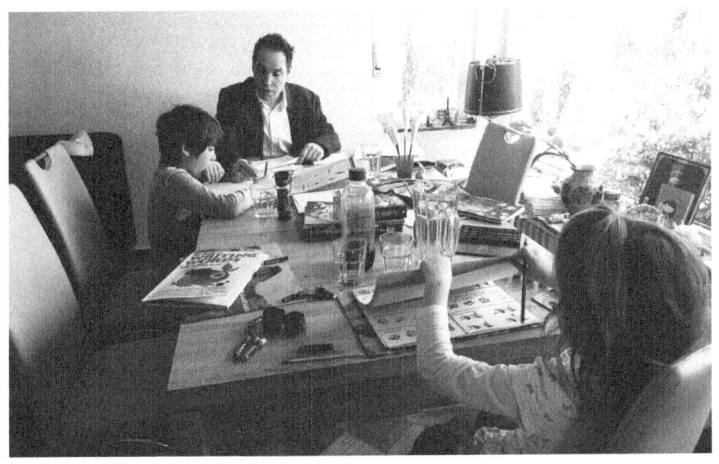

Home schooling took over from regular schooling in many countries creating "working from home" difficulties for the parents

INDIA: MIGRANT WORKERS

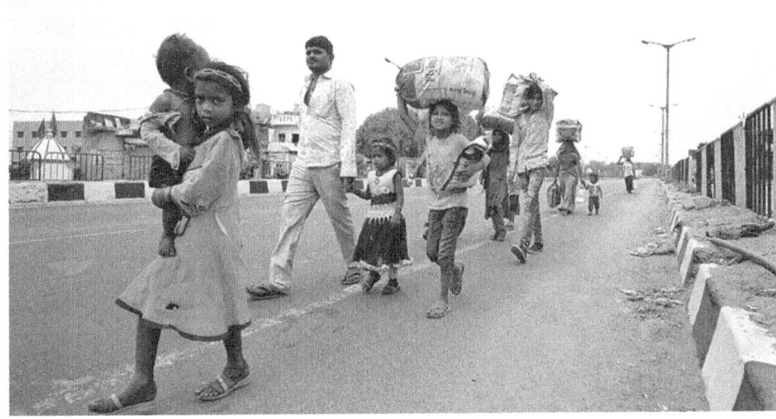

In India the lockdown due to COVID-19 caused loss of jobs for thousands of migrant workers who walked back to their villages hundreds of miles way. There was no rail or bus during the strict lockdown days. ©public domain
Picture sent by Dr Arvind Chaturvedi

DEMONSTRATIONS IN THE USA

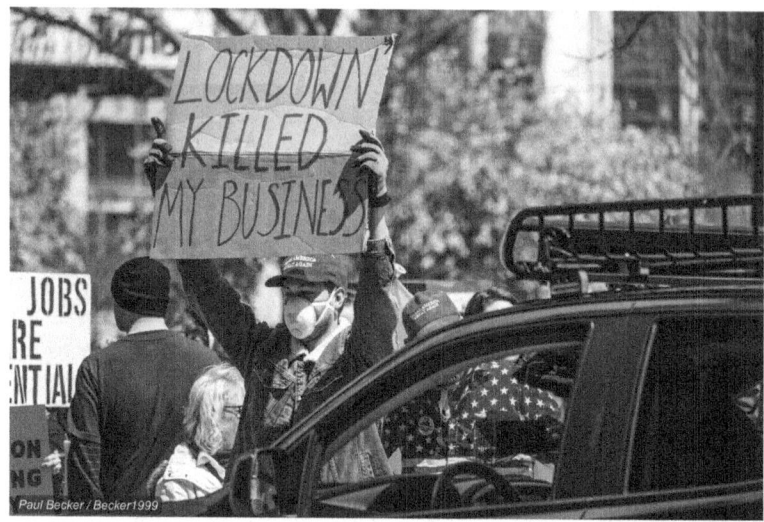

Above: *The United States of America, the land of the free, did not take kindly to lockdown. From mid-April there were protests organised by right wing groups against the restriction of business activity and the curtailing of freedom.*
Below: *In May the murder of George Floyd by police officer Derek Chauvin sparked riots and protests worldwide. A protester stands on a police car with a smashed windowshield outside the Target in the Midway area of St Paul, Minnesota* (Author:Lorie Shaull from St Paul, United States This file is licensed under the Creative Commons via wikipedia)

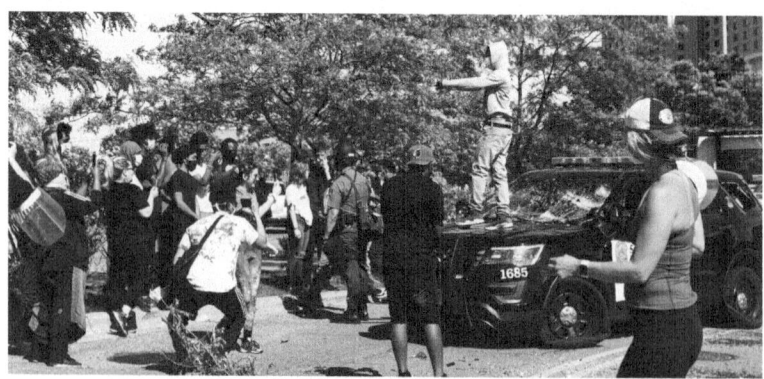

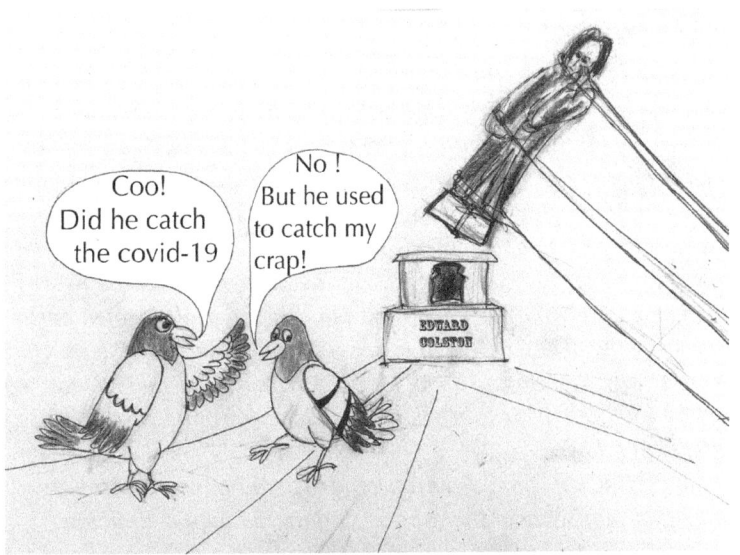

In the centre of Bristol UK riots sparked by the Black Lives Matter campaign led to Edward Colston's statue being toppled and thrown into the docks. Colston had been a slaver who put a considerable portion of his wealth into charitable work

Excess deaths

The adverse effects of COVID-19 were described in chapter 12. The default response in most countries was to lockdown the populace. Some of the the adverse effects of lockdown are re-iterated or described for the first time in this chapter.

In Chapter 12 excess deaths were documented in the community and in nursing homes that were not due to COVID-19. It is my contention that these extra deaths were the result of lockdown, government legislation and propaganda.

A climate of fear and policies of isolation were engendered such that people were even afraid to visit relatives and talk to them through a closed window. The policy of staying away from hospitals and GPs in order to protect the NHS went too far and many people with significant and possibly life-threatening disease avoided seeking help. When they did go to hospital they were at some considerable risk of catching COVID-19 from the hospital staff and other patients! Older patients in hospital who were suspected of having COVID-19 were discharged into nursing homes where many died.

This is how I reported the phenomenon in the first issue of this book

"May 20th 2020 [1]

"The Blame Game has started. As the daily count of deaths begins to fall people are beginning to notice what is happening in the care homes. There the counts are rising. At the beginning of the lockdown two aims were put forward.... to flatten the curve and thus protect the NHS and to protect the most vulnerable. These were initially stated as being everyone over seventy then refined to be people who were on immunosuppressants, chemotherapy or very old and infirm. So surely that meant the care homes? Yet as soon as the crisis heated up the hospitals immediately put the care homes under pressure as noted earlier.

Labour's new leader, Sir Keir Starmer, asked at Prime Minister's Questions, "Government advice from 2nd to the 15th of April, was that and I quote, 'negative tests are not required prior to transfers or admissions into care homes'. What's protective about that?"

The Prime Minister Boris Johnson replied: "No one was discharged into a care home this year without the express authorisation of a clinician."

Not exactly answering the question.

Professor Stephen Powis, national medical director of NHS England, was asked later at a Downing Street briefing if the PM was passing the blame to doctors and replied:

"I'm absolutely sure that my medical colleagues would not be discharging patients under any circumstances unless they were sure that their medical treatment in hospital was complete, they were fit for discharge, and it was safe to discharge them." Which clearly was not the case as the discharged patients definitely seeded the nursing homes with COVID-19.

In my own experience hospital trusts around the country would have responded variably when asked to clear the wards. Having been told that negative tests are not required prior to transfers or admissions into care homes some managers would put the medics under pressure to clear the wards. In my time as a hospital doctor some trusts had a very poor record when worried about bed occupancy and did discharge patients too early. One obvious example that showed this was readmission to hospital following too early discharge after surgery.

It is clear that the management in some hospitals do insist that medical staff (including doctors, nurses, physiotherapists and occupational therapists) discharge patients against the medics' best judgement. Many are too scared to disagree and afraid that if they speak up about it they will be "disciplined". Which is a thin disguise for legally sanctioned bullying of staff. We all know what being "disciplined" meant under the Soviet or Nazi regimes and, in my humble opinion, that is how the Human Resources departments behave.

So please don't blame the medical staff. Blame the directives that have come from above, blame the people who actually sanctioned them and blame the far-too-powerful management. Which is probably to suggest that Professor Stephen Powis, national medical director of NHS England, and his direct team should be the people questioned about this. Culture Secretary Oliver Dowden was asked if the issue of care homes had been glossed over.

"It is categorically not the case that we have glossed over this," he replied adding. "In any public health crisis like this there'll be a time for lessons to be learned afterwards."

It might be more useful if they learnt some of the lessons as the crisis unfolds."

And now in the Summer of 2021:

The Office for National Statistics (ONS) [2,3,4] reported that 41% of the excess deaths in England during the first lockdown were the result of missed medical care. This shows that 16,000 extra people died because of the lockdown substantiating my comments in Chapter 12 and my indictments in the first edition of PANDEMIC. Non-Covid deaths in March and April 2020 were 15.3% above the 5 year average but between May and July were 6% below, presumably due to deaths 'brought forward' in March and April. Deaths in private homes were still above average. The deaths in hospital had fallen to below average at this time indicating that too few patients were being treated in hospital.

Lung [5-9]: Twenty percent of deaths in the UK are due to lung diseases, including asthma, chronic obstructive pulmonary disease or other long term respiratory illness. Usually 10,000 people in the UK are newly diagnosed with a lung disease every week and at least half of these need to be immediately put on treatment. During the initial lockdown the NHS closed the clinics and emptied the wards, mostly into nursing homes. Patients found it very hard to access their GPs and diagnoses were made over the telephone.

Referrals of patients needing urgent care for lung conditions dropped by as much as 70% during lockdown in the UK. An average of 3,399 patients per week missed out on urgent and routine referrals during lockdown, according to the Taskforce for Lung Health and, due to long waiting lists, the access has continued to be poor. The data from NHS England, analysed by the Taskforce, also showed that nearly forty percent of Clinical Commissioning Groups (CCGs) in England did not see a single appointment booking for respiratory conditions in May, and 65% of CCGs had 5 or less bookings. Many thousands of patients with lung diseases have had delayed appointments and treatment. Conditions such as fibrosing alveolitis, where the lungs become progressively scarred with fibrosis, can result in a very short life expectancy and a delay in diagnosis can result in the patient missing out on significant treatment and support in the short period that they have left to live.

Respiratory function studies can induce coughing so their use has been suspended during the pandemic.

Sleep apnoea patients are often treated with CPAP devices and initial concerns that these may spread the Covid disease caused a drop in their use in March and April 2020. Subsequently the patients realised that this was only very rarely a problem and that CPAP may, in fact, help protect them, thus they continued to carefully follow their treatment regimes. The major concern now is the delay in diagnosing the condition and thus delays in starting treatment.

Smoking and Drinking. [10] "The first COVID-19 lockdown in England in March-July 2020 was associated with increased smoking prevalence among younger adults, and increased prevalence of high-risk drinking among all sociodemographic groups". This is the first time for years that smoking has increased and it will lead to increased morbidity and mortality from lung disease, primarily chronic obstructive airways disease and cancer. Increased alcohol intake will result in an increase in liver disease, neurological problems, cardiomyopathy, obesity and cancer.

Heart.[10,11] Data on cardiology referral rates showed those experiencing heart problems had much more access to care than lung patients, with just 1 in 5 (26%) of CCGs showing no bookings for cardiology, and 38% with 5 or less bookings in May.[10] However research published by the British Heart Foundation in July 2020 estimated that 5000 heart attack sufferers may have missed out on life saving hospital treatment due to the shut down of many hospital facilities and the urge to stay at home.

Obesity. [12-15] The condition of being morbidly overweight carries considerable health risks and major costs for the NHS and social services. Health risks range from coronary heart disease to cancer, mental illness to high blood pressure.

There is almost no common cause of death in the developed world which is not more frequent in obese people compared with those of normal weight. Unfortunately the UK was seeing a major increase in obesity before the COVID-19 pandemic. Due to the lockdown this problem has markedly worsened. A study published in October 2020 looked at the eating behaviour and physical activity during COVID-19 lockdown. Over two thousand adults completed a survey and this showed that a large number showed worsening of eating habits and exercise behaviour during the first lockdown. For example well over half the respondents reported snacking more frequently. People who were already overweight or obese reported even lower levels of physical activity and diet quality, and a greater reported frequency of overeating.

People on a low income are at a greater risk of obesity, eat worse food and exercise less. This has worsened due to lockdowns that impact their income and thus the quality of their food and prevent them from doing inexpensive exercise.

In fact the double whammy of closing businesses and public facilities such as parks and swimming pools particularly affects those who are the most socially deprived. Obesity doubles the risk of dying from COVID-19 so preventing people from doing the things that might have reduced that risk does seem absurd. Whilst one hour a day of exercise was permitted it is hard to understand why any limit was set. People were arrested for resting alone on a bench when out exercising and when sunbathing on their own. This problem does not just affect the adult population. In the UK one in three children are leaving primary school overweight and one in five are living with obesity.

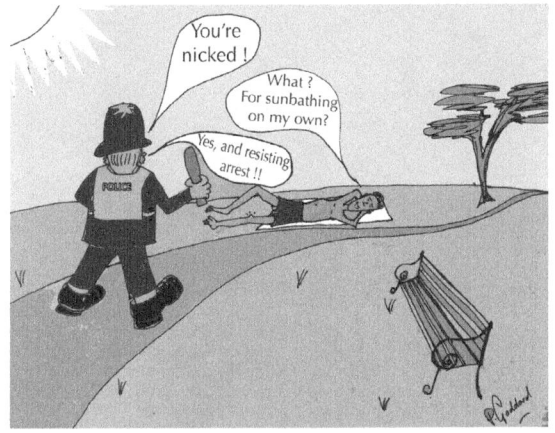

Type 2 Diabetes. [16-19] Ninety percent of the cases of Type 2 Diabetes are related to obesity. According to reports from the virtual Diabetes UK Professional Conference the lockdown has been a disaster with regard to the diagnosis and treatment of diabetes. This is not surprising since only a third of patients could access the NHS in the first wave. Matthew Carr Research Fellow, University of Manchester, presenting at the virtual conference, stated that in the first wave of COVID-19 the diagnosis rate of type 2 diabetes and new prescriptions for the preferred treatment, metformin, fell by 70% in April. Given that obesity levels are soaring with two thirds of adults already overweight or obese and the levels rising during lockdown, this represents a frighteningly serious figure. Over the period March to December more than a quarter of the diabetes cases were missed. Carr reported that "our estimate of 60,000 missed or delayed diagnoses may well be an underestimate if changes in lifestyle during the pandemics and lockdowns have increased obesity rates of other risk factors for diabetes in the general population."

Delayed diagnosis leads to the condition of the patients deteriorating before they are finally treated thus increasing the burden on the patients and the health service and increasing the death toll!

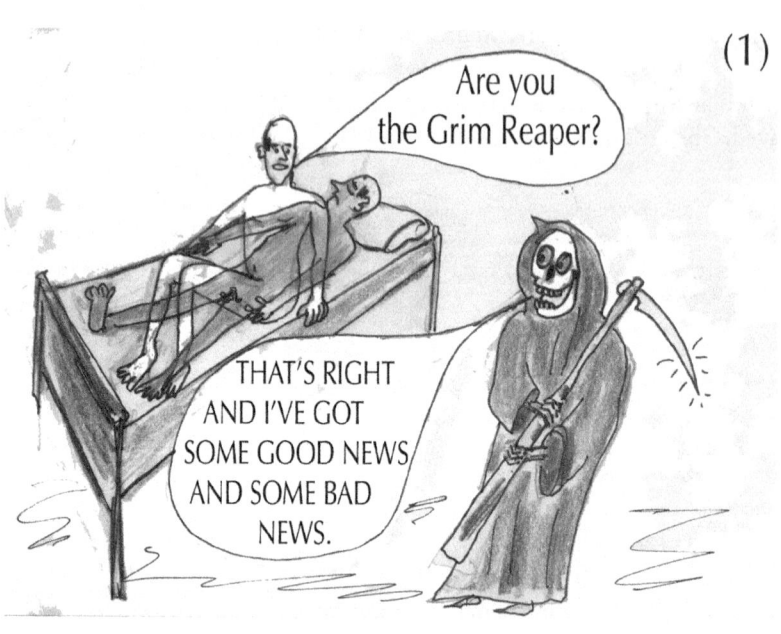
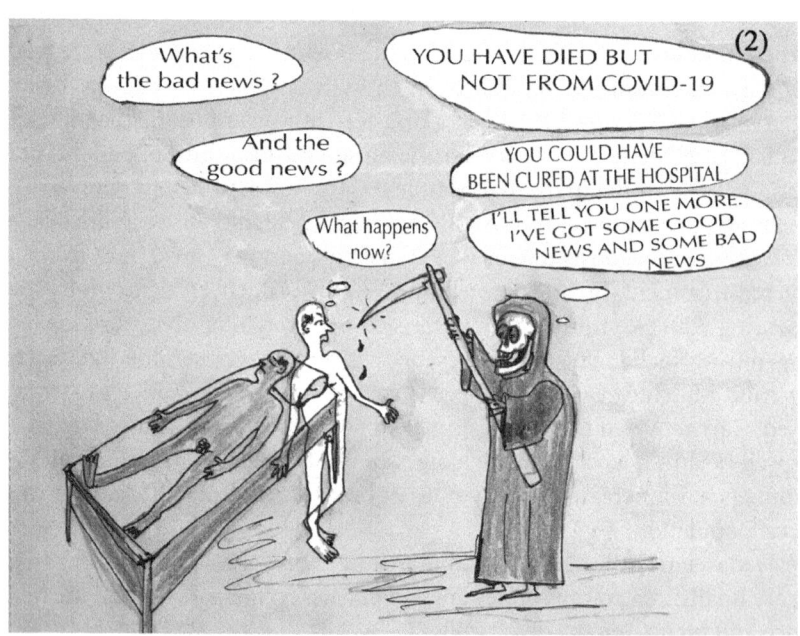

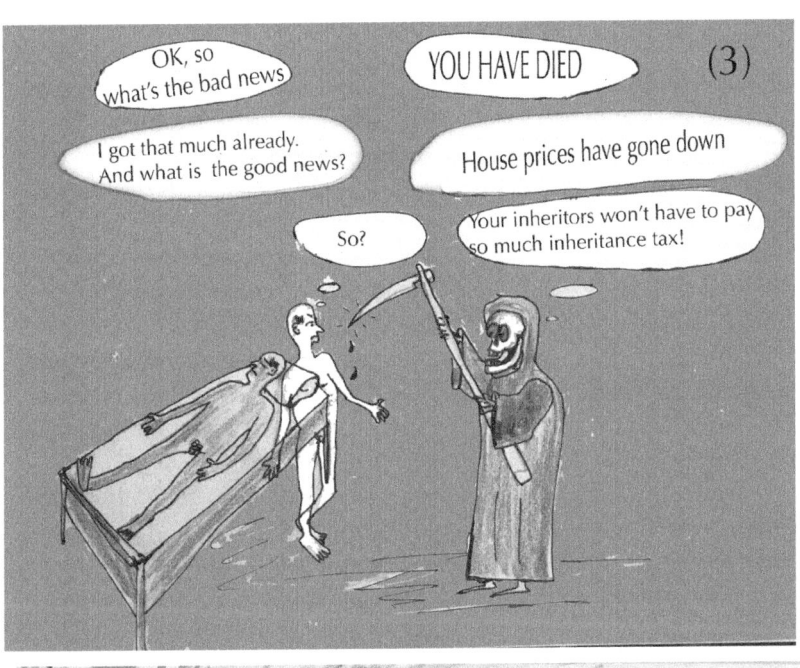
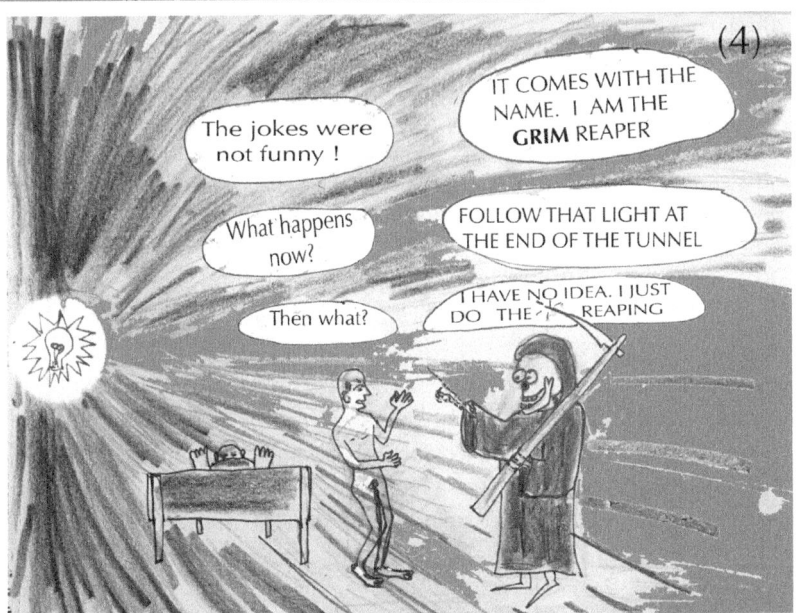

Richard Batterham Professor of Obesity, Diabetes and Endocrinology, University College London and Steve Bain, Professor of Medicine (Diabetes), Swansea University, speaking at the same conference, referred to the enormous backlog problem in the world of COVID and lockdowns and the barriers facing overweight patients with regard to treatment. These barriers included lack of services in deprived areas, stigma, impact of COVID, and patient psychology/empowerment to navigate NHS systems. All the problems had been made worse by lockdowns.

According to the Mayo clinic the symptoms of untreated type 2 diabetes are myriad. Diabetes commonly affects many major organs. In the cardiovascular system it causes heart disease, stroke and high blood pressure. Nerve damage, kidney disease, eye damage, hearing impairment and dementia are also increased in incidence. Diabetes increases susceptibility to skin infections and low healing of cuts and blisters. Severe damage may require toe, foot or leg amputation.

Early treatment reduces the risks associated with diabetes and delayed diagnosis is therefore a major problem. The supposed benefits of lockdowns should have been weighed against the major drawbacks and safeguards put in place to ensure that conditions such as diabetes did not go undiagnosed. This was not done.

Case A

A 73 year-old man with known Type II diabetes suffered from loss of vision in his eye. Because of lockdown an appointment with his GP was considerably delayed but the doctor considered the condition needed urgent referral for ophthalmic care. The eye appointment was, however, delayed for 5 months during which the patient experienced considerable difficulties due to double vision. Eventually at the appointment a diagnosis of retinal/ vitreous detachment and haemorrhage was made. Urgent treatment was suggested but the eye doctors were not able to see him again to undertake the treatment for another few months. Eventually the double vision improved but vision in one eye continued to be poor. No actual treatment was undertaken.

Cancer: As discussed above the increased smoking, increased alcohol consumption and increased obesity all lead to an increased incidence of cancer. Obesity has now overtaken smoking as the most common predisposing factor for cancer. This is compounding the effects of lockdown where many patients were forced to miss appointments and some treatments were simply stopped. The initial diagnosis of cancer has been delayed in many patients.

Overall by August 2020 it was predicted that an additional 18,000 deaths from cancer will result from the pandemic and the response to it.

Mental health. [20-40] The COVID-19 pandemic has affected mental health in a myriad of ways. There has been the direct effect on health due to infection, the effects on people forcibly kept away from work and from friends and family by lockdowns, shielding and self-isolation, the uncertainty about future employment and the possibility or not of returning to work. In addition the effects of the pandemic on the mental health of clinical staff and frontline workers should not be ignored and is likely to be very significant.

The Public

The Lockdown resulted in large numbers of people having uncertainty over their jobs (especially with the second lockdown), losing daytime activity, and either being socially isolated or having to spend protracted periods of time with their family. All of these are associated with increased mental morbidity.

A recent study has shown that separation anxiety is an important factor in assessing suicide risk. Pini et al found that their study *'indicates a substantial role of separation anxiety in predicting suicidal thoughts, both as state-related symptoms (evaluated by HDRS item 3) and as longitudinal dimensional symptoms (as evaluated by MOODS-SR). Greater understanding of the influence of separation anxiety in patients with affective disorders may encourage personalized interventions for reducing suicide risk.'*

Previous studies have cited separation anxiety in children and adolescents as a risk factor for suicide but this study highlighted its importance in adults

The study was undertaken before the advent of the COVID-19 pandemic but does bring into question the wisdom of the punitive level of separation brought in by the lockdowns in many countries.

In the UK adherence to the policy of self-isolation has been high (data from the Office of National Statistics discussed in Medscape). But with the reported 82% adherence the survey also stated that the self-isolation had worsened wellbeing and mental health in 35% and 28% had lost income.

The stress of the pandemic and the restrictions has worsened the nation's smoking habits with 30% of smokers smoking more regularly and 10% of those who had given up starting again!

In Japan an initial small drop in suicide rates of 14% during the first wave of the pandemic was followed by a small rise of 16% during the second wave.

COVID-19 itself can have severe effects on the neurological system and a difficulty in thinking, known as 'brain fogging', is a common symptom during Covid infection and as a symptom of "long Covid". Brain fog and headache have also been reported as relatively common side-effects following vaccination.

Lockdowns have increased anxiety amongst all age groups. Some 20% of people are worried about going back to work at the end of lockdown and 23% worried about public transport. The climate of fear engendered to persuade people to self-isolate, lockdown and submit themselves to vaccination has also created a heightened level of anxiety.

Many people in England have welcomed the end of lockdown and the chance of returning to a restaurant or pubs but a substantial minority are worried about resuming social contact.

All of the harmful effects of lockdown have been far worse for people on low income and living in inadequate housing. It is one thing for the privileged few to self-isolate whilst on a decent pension and living in a large detached house with a garden and quite another to be forced to work due to lack of income yet finding that this is almost impossible because the children are at home in a one bedroomed flat. Add to that not being allowed to even sit down on a bench in the local park and after all this getting symptoms of COVID-19 and not being allowed to see the family practitioner because she is shielding herself! Is this a true scenario? In lockdowns you bet it is!

Case B
A man aged 21, working as a heating engineer, had suffered from anxiety in the past. 'The lockdowns have made it a million times worse. A friend committed suicide in the first lockdown and I sat on the same bridge wondering whether it was worth going on. I didn't have the nerve to kill myself but I understood why he did it. I just felt that I couldn't inflict my suicide on my parents and brother. I get some relief now by going to the gym, putting on my headphones and getting into the zone. I'm not going out at all apart from working. I have to work as there would be no money coming in otherwise and my work is considered as an essential service. I'm afraid of meeting people in a social situation.'

Children and Adolescents

The COVID-19 pandemic has only rarely caused severe infection in children and the main cause of concern has been the effects of lockdown and isolation on their mental health. After several weeks of the first lockdown in April 2020 a child of infant school age was overheard plaintively enquiring: 'Mummy, why don't I have any friends anymore?'

The playgrounds in the park were barred and the swings padlocked. Adolescents climbed over to use the remaining equipment and adults with young children stood impotently around with younger children who were complaining that it was unfair: 'Why can the old children use the playground and we can't?'

The Daily Telegraph reports that mental health referrals for children rose considerably in 2020 with 1 in 9 experiencing mental health problems in 2017 rising to 1 in 6 by mid 2020.

Moreover due to the very real worries about the vaccines it is unlikely that children can expect vaccination to free them as it has the adults.

Health Workers and other frontline staff

Whilst many of the public have been furloughed and only working intermittently during the pandemic the experience of the health workers and frontline staff in essential jobs has been very different. Many of these people, such as care assistants in nursing homes and shop assistants, are amongst the lowest paid people in our society but are essential for its continuance. They have had to endure long working hours dressed in cumbersome, uncomfortable and often ineffective personal protective equipment (PPE).

In addition to this health workers have to face the threat of infection which, due to the potentially high viral load, may prove fatal. Also many health workers have co-morbidities, such as chronically low vitamin D, obesity and sickle cell trait, that make them susceptible to COVID-19.

In the first lockdown the uncertainties over treatment protocols, the shortage of PPE and the absence of nearly all the usual patients, led to considerable anxiety amongst hospital and nursing home staff. Patients were discharged into nursing homes in the UK without proper testing and the staff receiving them were soon in great difficulties. Throughout the healthcare sector staff levels have been historically low because of staff, by necessity, self-isolating every time they had a slight cold or sniffle. Lack of testing initially was a factor in worsening the anxiety levels and some have rejected vaccination due to concerns over the safety of the vaccines,

The lockdowns decreased the number of patients with complaints other than COVID-19 being seen and treated in the hospitals. Now the NHS staff have to cope with the enormous backlog of 4.7 million people waiting to start treatment on the NHS in England alone. That was the figure at the end of February 2021 and is the highest figure since records began in 2007. The President of the Royal College of Physicians (RCP), Professor Andrew Goddard, recently called for a doubling of the number of doctors in the UK. The RCP stated that *"Globally, more than 300,000 health-care workers have been infected with COVID-19 in 79 countries, over 7,000 have died, and many more have suffered as a result of stress, burnout, and moral injury."*

Dementia , Learning Difficulties and Disablements

Patients with dementia and people with learning difficulties have been shown to be particularly at risk during the lockdowns. Their life expectancy has worsened due not only to the COVID-19 but also due to isolation. According to one care home owner: 'Without the visits from family and friends and the hands-on support from the care home staff many of the dementia sufferers have lost the will to live and simply died.'

Dementia sufferers in the community and those with learning disabilities find it very hard to cope with the new restrictions and are bewildered by the lack of interaction from family and friends. They also find the more stringent hygiene regimes difficult to follow. This may, in turn make them more liable to infection.

The deaf find it impossible to lip-read when people are wearing masks and blind people are unable to read many of the new notices about restrictions in shops, such as a refusal to take cash (card only sales).

Speaking to one disabled person who has very restricted mobility we were told: 'When the first lockdown came I was inexplicably not classed as vulnerable despite my disabilities. I was at the back of the queue when trying to get a delivery slot for food online and, when I was almost out of food in my flat, the delivery man refused to carry the items up to my landing due to fear of catching the Covid. My physical health deteriorated because I was not allowed to visit the swimming pool for aquatic therapy. The overall effect of lockdown was very detrimental.'

UK Politicians

Perhaps bravado informed the UK politicians in the first few weeks of the pandemic when they did nothing and assumed we would simply avoid being affected as had been the case with SARS1, MERS and Ebola. Now fear of new variants, fear of being too lenient and fear of incriminations appears to be the dominant feature in Downing Street. As the Daily Telegraph stated 'If a fear of vaccine-resistant variants is now driving policy it is hard to see how normal life can resume.' There has been no effective opposition to the draconian measures brought in by the UK government. The official leader of the opposition, Labour leader Sir Kier Starmer, has shown his true colours by consistently asking Boris Johnson to make the restrictions more severe. His point has been that most people agree with the lockdowns and restrictions. As an article by Jonathan Sumpton states: 'When democracy becomes a mechanism for mass coercion, with the approval of the opposition, it is surely heading towards its end.'

Many people have been shocked by a recent revelation that many of the top civil servants have appointments with industry that surely provide a conflict of interest. Already on very high salaries they have taken up these jobs whilst still employed in the civil service! Bureaucratic dictatorship really is taking over in the UK.

General comments about socialising

The longterm detrimental effects of the lockdowns can presently only be guessed but the health benefits of socialising are well known so the absence of social interaction is bound to have enormous detrimental effect.

Important beneficial effects of socialising include improvement in mental health and decrease in depression. Good social interaction boosts confidence and self-esteem. People who are lonely often have low confidence and esteem. Loneliness correlates with functional decline and is a risk factor for high blood pressure. Social isolation increases the risk of Alzheimer's. According to Wilson et al "Risk of Alzheimer's Disease was more than doubled in lonely persons compared with persons who were not lonely."

Being sociable boosts immunity and has other physical health benefits. Socialization can reduce the risk for cardiovascular disease, cancer, osteoporosis, and rheumatoid arthritis.

Socialisation boosts cognitive function and spending time with others helps us feel useful and that our life has a purpose so, conversely, being forced into isolation may have the opposite effect. There is some evidence that the first lockdown did not adversely affect mental health very badly as people felt that it would only be for a short time and the we were "all in it together." Subsequent lockdowns have eroded that sense of purpose and various advisers and politicians who have broken the rules that they have imposed on everybody else have managed to make the public very annoyed and wonder why they are having to obey the seemingly arbitrary regulations.

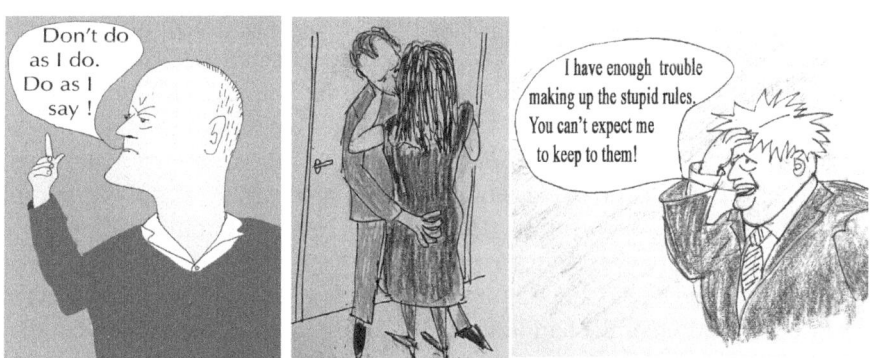

Dominic Cummings, Hancock and Boris all liked to flaunt the rules. Cummings and Hancock have gone but Boris remains.

The pandemic has resulted in multiple causes of concern with regard to mental health and these have been compounded by the draconian lockdowns and their enforcement. COVID-19 infection can cause long term brain fog and depression and these effects are worsened by the lockdowns. Human beings are social animals and being forced into isolation is used in prison as a very severe form of punishment. Now, however, completely innocent people are being put into nursing homes and denied contact with their families for extended periods. During lockdowns people cannot visit theatres, cinemas, taverns, churches and even the accommodation of friends. The general misery this has created will be transferred into an increased incidence of mental and physical illness. Indeed recent research, widely reported in the media shows the incidence of significant depression in adults more than doubling over the past year and affecting nearly a quarter of the population. Lockdown and self-isolation may cause separation anxiety and the vaccines, despite claims to the contrary, do have a high incidence of side-effects including headache and confusion. Suicide has shown an upswing in the second wave and subsequent lockdowns.

Healthcare staff are at considerable risk of stress, burnout and injury. Dementia sufferers have had their lives shortened by COVID-19 but more so by the lockdowns. Meanwhile the UK politicians seem to be making decisions based on fear and the civil servants have given up their right to claim impartiality by taking on appointments with industry.

Education

School

Back at school the children had to remain in 'bubbles' and wear masks. As soon as they left school each day they played together in the parks showing that the wearing of masks is not to protect themselves but perhaps to pacify the teachers.

The long period away from school means that the youngest children have not had the important socialisation effects of pre-school and the infant schools. Schools help to teach children what is expected of them as they mature and become full members of society. Older children have missed significant education and the opportunity of doing their best in examinations and talk of a 'lost generation' has only served to make them even more anxious about their future. Home schooling has at best been very patchy and the worst affected have been children of the families with the lowest incomes but even in families with high income the effect on education and mental health has been striking. Parents who have to undertake home schooling cannot, at the same time, work from home. Naturally the more children in the family the more stress home schooling brings to the family unit. In the UK nearly 15% of families are lone parent families which markedly adds to the stress when asked to home school.

Globally the lockdowns and concomitant school closures have impacted more than 1.5 billion children. According to the WHO: 'Movement restrictions, loss of income, isolation, overcrowding and high levels of stress and anxiety are increasing the likelihood that children experience and observe physical, psychological and sexual abuse at home – particularly those children already living in violent or dysfunctional family situations.'

In the UK reports are circulating that 20,000 pupils are missing from the roll call now that the students are back at school. There is no official register of children being homeschooled and it is not known how many of the missing children are having schooling or have simply stopped being taught.

The "madness" of constantly testing and isolating children has sparked considerable concern. Why is the testing and isolation being done and who are the authorities trying to protect? Clearly if the COVID-19 only mildly affects children this is not being done to protect them, thus it must have been introduced to protect adults such as teachers, parents and relatives. This is at considerable cost to the children. One parent described how her child had seven times been sent home to isolate along a with all the other members of the "bubble" because one child tested positive. A friend told me that her child and ninety other children had been barred from a school walk because one child tested positive on a lateral flow test. The PCR test proved negative so the entire outing had been cancelled due to a false positive test.

The schemes to reduce spread of COVID-19 in schools have included keeping within socially distanced hoops, sanitising books, surrounding desks with black and yellow tape and constant mask-wearing, cancellation of exams and avoidance of practical subjects such as work in science laboratories. The mask-wearing can lead to physical problems such as skin, mouth, throat and chest infections and the social isolation is like a very tough punishment. In addition wearing most types of mask leads to an increased level of carbon dioxide since the expired air is not completely dissipated when the mask wearer inhales. This is akin to respiratory acidosis seen, for example, in patients with chronic lung diseases such a chronic bronchitis and also observed in people with sleep apnoea.

Schoolchildren are being forced to wear masks for hours on end and this is causing unacceptable levels of CO_2. According to Wallach et al writing in JAMA Pediatrics: *"The normal content of carbon dioxide in the open is about 0.04% by volume (ie, 400 ppm). A level of 0.2% by volume or 2000 ppm is the limit for closed rooms according to the German Federal Environmental Office, and everything beyond this level is unacceptable."* When wearing masks *"the value of the child with the lowest carbon dioxide level was 3-fold greater than the limit of 0.2 % by volume. The youngest children had the highest values, with one 7-year-old child's carbon dioxide level measured at 25,000 ppm."*

It is, in any case, totally ineffective since as soon as they are out of school the children meet up in the parks and play areas with no thought of isolating or mask-wearing……..and why should they isolate? The measures were not brought in to help the children and many of them are fully aware of this.

University

The useful experience of University has always included the effect of meeting and socialising with the peer group and one-to-one discussions with the lecturers. In the UK the only courses that have permitted such interaction have been those with a practical element. All social events for new students starting in October 2020 were cancelled and for theoretical subjects only distance learning was permitted. An increase in students asking for help due to mental problems has occurred over the last few years and the Covid restrictions have exacerbated the problems.

The Test and Trace "Pingdemic"

The problems of test and trace were mentioned in chapter 12. As I write this the "freedom day" has come and gone but people are being "pinged" by the test and trace app when they have not left their home for days. They might, by virtue of their house being in a terrace or flat being in an apartment block, be close to other accommodation where a person has tested positive. By law they have to self-isolate unless they can prove that it is a false alarm. Stressful, nonsensical and time-wasting but very serious. Businesses are being closed by it and essential services (including the NHS) badly affected. Empty shelves in the supermarkets are witness to the fact that the supply chains are being affected by so many staff being forced to self-isolate. The Government has responded by offering exemptions. The unions have told workers to self-isolate and ignore the exemptions, thus making life worse.

Many hospital staff have deleted the app from their mobile phones. Others are following suit.

Economy

This book is not about economics but a discussion on the dire effects of COVID-19 and the Lockdowns would not be complete without a mention of the economy. The economic effects of closing businesses are obvious but need repeating. The government's furlough scheme was exceedingly expensive but incomplete. Many of the self-employed fell through the net and received no support. Some people who had been on higher incomes received no support. Many people were made redundant just before the furlough scheme started or were made redundant during the scheme because of the costs of the part that their employees had to bear. It has been suggested that the unemployment figures in the UK, which have been reported as 5%, do not reflect the true state of affairs. Almost two million people are in hidden unemployment: "They are out of work and eager to find jobs but are classified as economically inactive rather than unemployed"[5]. Clearly when children were not allowed to go to school one of the parents was very likely to have become "economically inactive".

The poorer people had a far worse experience of lockdown and many took to snacking, greater alcohol intake and increased smoking.

The hospital executives and some people on the SAGE committee (notably the Communist Professor Susan Michie) called for greater and longer lockdowns. The hospital chiefs did so on the grounds that there was an enormous backlog due to the previous lockdowns. Hence the Helterskelter to Hell cartoon below:

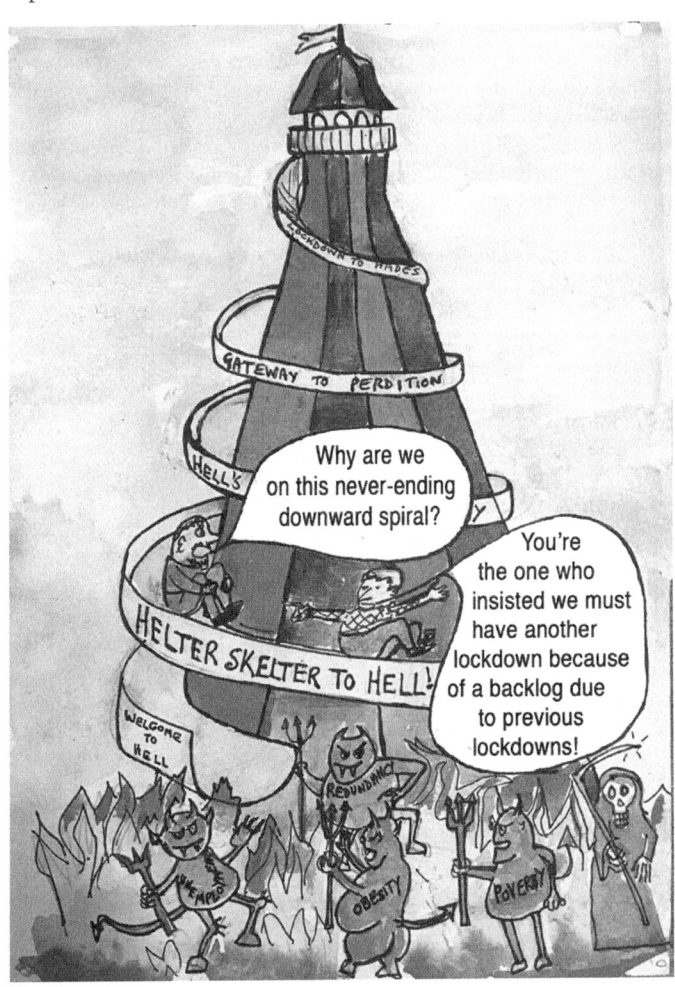

Luckily Boris resisted the clarion calls of the far left and the self-serving thoughts of the NHS chief executives and permitted increased freedom. Apart from the ongoing "pingdemic" the gamble appears to have paid off this time. The virus has not gone away and now that it exists we can expect more pandemics from it in the future but at the present the 4th wave is waning.

Some other countries have fared better economically. China, the country where it all started, came out of recession very quickly but governments around the world are becoming aware of the way that the Chinese Communist Party Government has behaved. As I write the news has broken that China is refusing to have another enquiry into the origin of the virus.

References

1. 1. Paul R Goddard PANDEMIC (1st Edition) Clinical Press June 2020
2. https://news.sky.com/story/coronavirus-lockdown-may-have-indirectly-caused-16-000-excess-deaths-study-12044923
3. https://www.ons.gov.uk/peoplepopulationandcommunity/birthsdeathsandmarriages/deaths/articles/analysisofdeathregistrationsnotinvolvingcoronaviruscovid19englandandwales28december2019to1may2020/28december2019to10july2020#causes-of-non-COVID-19-deaths
4. https://statistics.blf.org.uk/
5. https://www.ons.gov.uk/peoplepopulationandcommunity/birthsdeathsandmarriages/deaths/articles/analysisofdeathregistrationsnotinvolvingcoronaviruscovid19englandandwales28december2019to1may2020/28december2019to10july2020#causes-of-non-COVID-19-deaths
6. https://www.blf.org.uk/taskforce/get-in-touch/media/patients-needing-urgent-care-for-lung-conditions
7. https://digital.nhs.uk/dashboards/ers-open-data.
8. https://www.gov.uk/government/publications/respiratory-disease-applying-all-our-health/respiratory-disease-applying-all-our-health
9. https://www.sleepreviewmag.com/sleep-treatments/therapy-devices/cpap-pap-devices/COVID-19-pandemic-insomnia-cpap-use-sleep-apnea-osa/
10. https://www.news-medical.net/news/20210218/Changes-in-drinking-and-smoking-during-Englande28099s-first-COVID-19-lockdown.aspx
11. https://www.blf.org.uk/taskforce/get-in-touch/media/patients-needing-urgent-care-for-lung-conditions
12. https://www.cdc.gov/obesity/adult/causes.html
13. Obesity, eating behavior and physical activity during COVID-19 lockdown: A study of UK adults EricRobinsonEmmaBoylandAnnaChisholmJoanneHarroldNiamh G.Maloney-LucileMartyBethan R.MeadRobNoonanCharlotte A.Hardman https://www.sciencedirect.com/science/article/abs/pii/S0195666320310060?via%3Dihub)
14. Fears grow of nutritional crisis in lockdown UK BMJ 2020; 370 doi: https://doi.org/10.1136/bmj.m3193
15. https://www.cancer.gov/about-cancer/causes-prevention/risk/obesity/obesity-fact-sheet#what-is-known-about-the-relationship-between-obesity-and-cancer-
16. Quarter of diabetes cases missed over lockdown as obesity soars: Daily Telegraph 26.4.2021

17. Only a third could access the NHS Daily Telegraph 26.4.2021
18. Indirect effects of COVID-19 pandemic on type 2 diabetes diagnosis and monitoring across the UK Matthew Carr. Virtual Diabetes UK Professional Conference 2021
19. https://www.mayoclinic.org/diseases-conditions/type-2-diabetes/symptoms-causes/syc-20351193
20. https://www.psychiatrist.com/jcp/depression/separation-anxiety-measures-of-suicide-risk-among-patients-mood-anxiety-disorders/?utm_source=jcp-gl&utm_medium=email&utm_campaign=jcp040121a&utm_content=20m13299&mc_cid=45c5443ce3&mc_eid=84ed32a4c0 Pini S, Abelli M, Costa B, et al. Separation anxiety and measures of suicide risk among patients with mood and anxiety disorders. J Clin Psychiatry. 2021;82(2):20m13299
21. chttps://www.medscape.com/viewarticle/949020?src=WNL_infoc_210416_MSCPEDIT_Markle&uac=285238SV&impID=3314037&faf=1#vp_2
22. https://www.medscape.com/viewarticle/949324?src=wnl_newsalrt_uk_210415_MSCPEDIT&uac=285238SV&impID=3313417&faf=1#vp_2
23. Tanaka, T., Okamoto, S. Increase in suicide following an initial decline during the COVID-19 pandemic in Japan. Nat Hum Behav 5, 229–238 (2021). https://doi.org/10.1038/s41562-020-01042-z
24. https://www.healthline.com/health/covid-brain-fog
25. https://www.nytimes.com/2020/12/28/us/vaccine-first-patients-covid.html
26. Thomson H, Why going back to offices may affect mental health, New Scientist 17 April 2021 p10
27. https://www.who.int/news/item/08-04-2020-joint-leader-s-statement---violence-against-children-a-hidden-crisis-of-the-COVID-19-pandemic#:~:text=The%20situation%20is%20aggravated%20by,marriage%20and%20child%20trafficking.
28. https://www.mirror.co.uk/news/uk-news/20000-kids-missing-school-amid-23966700
29. https://www.theguardian.com/education/2018/jun/21/thousands-of-pupils-missing-from-english-school-rolls-study
30. https://www.healthline.com/health/respiratory-acidosis#symptoms
31. https://jamanetwork.com/journals/jamapediatrics/fullarticle/2781743
32. Experimental Assessment of Carbon Dioxide Content in Inhaled Air With or Without Face Masks in Healthy Children A Randomized Clinical Trial. Harald Walach, PhD1; Ronald Weikl, MD2; Juliane Prentice, BA3; et al
33. We need a plan to fix the NHS backlog. Editorial comment. Daily Telegraph Friday 16 April 2021 https://www.rcplondon.ac.uk/news/rcp-calls-urgent-measures-protect-and-safeguard-medical-workforce
34. Daily Telegraph, Editorial, 20 April 2021
35. Jonathan Sumpton : Starmer betrayed a chilling truth about lockdown. Daily Telegraph, 21 April 2021
36. https://www.thetimes.co.uk/article/civil-servants-must-disclose-outside-work-as-greensill-scandal-widens-qcvrbqjnc
37. https://homecareassistance.com/blog/health-benefits-of-socialization
38. Robert S Wilson 1, Kristin R Krueger, Steven E Arnold, Julie A Schneider, Jeremiah F Kelly, Lisa L Barnes, Yuxiao Tang, David A Bennett Loneliness and risk of Alzheimer disease Arch Gen Psychiatry 2007 Feb;64(2):234-40.doi: 10.1001/archpsyc.64.2.234.
39. https://www.medscape.com/viewarticle/944943?src=WNL_ukmdpls_210508mscpedit_gen&uac=285238SV&impID=3358561&faf=1
40. https://www.thetimes.co.uk/article/two-million-hidden-unemployed-are-masking-true-cost-of-the-pandemic-wrfznsrcm

Chapter 15
Treatments for COVID-19

(including repurposed drugs and vitamins)

When the pandemic started there was much pessimism about treatment. Since the virus was completely new there were no drugs licensed for its treatment thus any pharmaceuticals used were repurposed drugs. By definition these are pharmaceuticals which have already previously been developed for use in human beings and are now used for a different purpose. For their original use they have already passed safety trials and are in use medically. They are frequently outside the patent time which is usually twenty years from initial time of filing with the patents office and they are therefore cheap and not profitable for the drug companies.

However, the Chief Medical Officer (CMO) in the UK instructed clinicians that they should not use repurposed drugs until trials had shown whether or not they were effective. But COVID-19 although a new virus was not a completely unknown entity. In broad terms it is a respiratory infection that leads to pneumonia and organ failure, something that can happen with many respiratory infections including influenza, Legionnaire's disease, pneumococcal infection and even measles. More specifically it is very similar to SARS (Severe Acute Respiratory Syndrome) and MERS (Middle East Respiratory Syndrome).

With the knowledge of similarly presenting infections it was reasonable to assume that prophylaxis against such infections and treatment of the common sequelae of the infections may have mitigated against the worst effects of COVID-19.

In the event many of the possible procedures, techniques and medicines were not initially used in the UK because of the instructions from the Chief Medical Officer and the Secretary of State for Health and Social Care.

We contend that their use should have been permitted and would have saved lives. A full investigation into the advice given to the CMO and Secretary of State and the instructions given out by them is undoubtedly necessary. Moreover scientific discussion about the origins of the virus are necessary not in order to attribute blame but to prevent such occurrences in the future.

In this chapter* we will try to delineate the techniques and pharmaceuticals that can prevent and treat the COVID-19 and its sequelae.

* written by Paul R Goddard, Dr Nabil Jarad and Professor Angus Dalgleish

The debate: untreatable or treatable?

Ferner and Aronoson writing in the BMJ [1] implied that COVID-19 was untreatable and suggested we should wait for vaccines or drugs targeted for specific structures in the virus rather than old drugs repurposed. Creating vaccines and rolling them out has taken nearly a year. A few new drugs have appeared but are not yet available for treatment of the public and a couple of drugs are on trial in Israel. Over four million people have died in the meantime.

Drug group	Efficacy in Covid-19 infection
Anti-virals	moderately useful (large trial)
Antibiotics (eg azithromycin), Anti-malarials (hydroxychloroquine etc.)	no specific benefit (large trial)
Anti-inflammatory drugs: corticosteroids	very useful in the inflammatory stages with cytokine storm (large trial)
Anti-inflammatory drugs: NSAIDs	colchicine and aspirin are useful, Monoclonal antibodies (eg Tocilizumab) very useful (large trial)
Anti-testosterone	preventative in patients on treatment for prostatic cancer
Anticoagulants	useful in late stages with intravascular thrombosis
Anti-parasitic (Ivermectin)	strong clinical support
Neurologically active drugs: amantadine	clinical support in patients with CNS impairment
Oxygen	very useful particularly with corticosteroids
Plasma	no specific benefit (large trial)
Anti-histamines	preventative in patients on treatment for asthma
Vitamin D3	preventative in people on treatment for low vitamin D. May be useful in clinical cases of Covid-19.

Table 1 Types of Drugs that may be useful in COVID-19 infection.

In a rapid response letter to the BMJ in April 2020,[2] Goddard, Jarad and Dalgleish supported the trials but pleaded for clinicians to be allowed to use their discretion in patients not entered on trials. Since the Ferner and Aronoson article referred to Hydroxychloroquine (HCQ) we used that as an example. The drug is relatively safe and inexpensive and is used in the UK for treatment of arthritis. It was considered to be possibly useful on its own or with azithromycin (AZM). To counter the argument that COVID-19 was untreatable we cited the examples of Remdesivir, a drug developed for use against Ebola. Remdesivir had been reported as useful in later stages of Covid infection.

We suggested that by the stage that oxygen and ventilation were necessary IL-6 monoclonal antibodies used for Rheumatoid arthritis may be helpful. Tocilizumab is one such example.

We saw no conflict between enrolling patients in clinical trials and trying off-label HCQ, AZM, anti-viral drugs or anti-inflammatory agents in Covid patients who were not being entered on the trials. We have also advocated the use of Vitamin D3, social distancing including masks and breathing exercises (Facebook, Youtube and the first edition of PANDEMIC).

Since the BMJ letter in April a plethora of drugs have been put forward for use in COVID-19 and many trials have taken place.

Outcome from trials

Hydroxychloroquine (HCQ)

Small trials had shown some efficacy but the Recovery trial [3] (Oxford 5 June 2020) showed no clinical benefit from the use of Hydroxychloroquine. It may still be useful in the early stages of the disease [4].

A paper in the Lancet [5], published Jan 01 2021, in a study of 194,637 people already on Hydroxychloroquine showed no increased mortality but some increased morbidity.

So it probably has little benefit but does not pose a great risk if prescribed and controlled by medical staff. We therefore do not advise its use and other drugs are likely to be more beneficial.

Azithromycin (AZM) and Doxycycline

AZM is a macrolide antibiotic effective in the treatment of chronic obstructive pulmonary disease (COPD, COAD). But the NIHR Principle and Recovery trials [6,7] showed no benefit in early or severe Covid infection. Doxycycline also showed no benefit.

Antivirals

Remdesivir and baricitinib (an anti-inflammatory, JAk inhibitor) combination led to faster recovery (NEJM)[8]. Tocilizumab (monoclonal antibody) has also been included with success[9].

Favipiravir has been approved for use in Covid in a number of countries [10,11,12]. Acyclovir has action against Covid in vitro though it has not yet been studied clinically [13].

Anti-inflammatory drugs

Corticosteroids

"Dexamethasone reduces death in hospitalised patients with severe respiratory complications of COVID-19" University of Oxford 16 June 2020.[14]

A meta-analysis study by the WHO rapid evidence appraisal has shown that hydrocortisone is also effective in reducing mortality rate (REACT)[15].

But a textbook from 1972 (Davidson et al) stated that at the stage of peripheral circulatory failure due to viral pneumonia high doses of corticosteroids may be of some value [16] so this was already a known fact. Was a trial really necessary? Professor Landrey (lead of the RECOVERY trial) stated recently " Had we been prescribing this drug from February 2020 we would have saved 4000 lives". [17] We believe that thousands of patients in the UK were denied high dose steroids unneccessarily.

Non-steroidal anti-inflammatory drugs (NSAIDs)

All of the NSAIDs may be of value in COVID-19. Aspirin, Colchicine and Tocilizumab [18] in particular are proving to be useful in combatting the inflammatory stage of COVID-19 infection.

Oxygen

Hypoxaemia and silent anoxia are features of COVID-19 infection and are one of the reasons that COVID-19 infection at high altitudes was particularly severe. Some organisms that cause pneumonia prefer the upper zones of the lungs and appear to thrive in higher oxygen tension. Tuberculosis and some fungal diseases (such as coccidioidomycosis) are in this category and interestingly sufferers from tuberculosis used to be sent to the Alps to convalesce. Other pneumonias occur predominantly in the lower zones and "prefer" lower levels of oxygenation. COVID-19 appears to be one of the latter and thrived in the ski resorts. Organisms that grow in excessively low oxygenation can cause anaerobic infections occurring after trauma but rarely cause pneumonia. Treatment of hypoxaemia with oxygen is by far the "most frequently prescribed drug" [19].

"The aim of supplemental oxygen therapy in patients with COVID-19 disease

is to support adequate oxygenation for physiological processes while avoiding hyperoxaemia, which may be harmful". [20,21]

Ivermectin

Ivermectin is a commonly prescribed drug which is approved for the treatment of parasitic infections. Its use against COVID-19 has strong clinical support and in trials Ivermectin has resulted in a marked reduction of self-reported anosmia/hyposmia, a reduction of cough and a tendency to lower viral loads and lower IgG titers. [22]

Other drugs of potential value.

Other classes of drugs that are proving useful in COVID-19 infection include anti-coagulants and neurologically active drugs such as Amantadine.[23] This drug was used initially against influenza but has been found effective against neurological impairment from COVID-19. More recently Polish doctors Konrad Rejdak and Pawel Grieb observed that twenty-two patients taking amantadine or memantine for multiple sclerosis, Parkinson disease or cognitive impairment did not have clinical manifestations of COVID-19 after testing positive for severe acute respiratory syndrome coronavirus. Amantadine may be showing some benefit due to its arousal-enhancing effect. Impaired consciousness is a frequent CNS manifestation of COVID-19 infection and amantadine may be useful in combatting this.

Also possibly useful are anti-testosterone therapy though the harmful effects may outweigh any benefit [24], anti-histamines [25] and anti-diabetic agents [26].

In late stages of the disease there is a syndrome much like disseminated intra-vascular coagulation (DIC) which is probably occurring due to intravascular haemolysis. At this stage anti-coagulants are useful [27].

Anti-histamines hydroxyzine (Atarax), diphenhyrdamine (benadryl) and azelastine (nasal spray) reduced symptoms and signs of COVID-19 infection in nearly a quarter of a million Californian patients who were on the drugs for cold and allergy symptoms [28]. This is an example of a strong association however it is not proof of efficacy as a treatment in patients with COVID-19 who were not previously on the drug.

The same can be applied to anti-testosterone therapy and anti-diabetic agents. The efficacy in reducing the risk of infection does not necessarily mean that the agents will be useful in treatment, though indeed they may be.

Prevention

Vitamin D3

Most people in the Northern hemisphere lack vitamin D in the winter months. Older people frequently have chronically low levels of vitamin D. It is not only important in preventing rickets and osteomalacia but it also has a significant role in the human immune system. A Barcelona study showed it cut deaths by 60% when administered to patients with COVID-19 infection.[29]

This was a small study so its role in treatment is still debatable but as a preventative measure it is very important. [30] The dose recommended for the immune system is larger than that for the bones .... at least 2000 IU per day.

Oral hygiene

There is a link between poor oral hygiene and severe COVID-19 infection [31]

Diabetes and Obesity

Both Diabetes and Obesity are risk factors so their treatment or prevention is essential. Treat the diabetes, encourage exercise and promote weight control.

Silent anoxia, Co-morbidities

Prevention of silent anoxia by using a pulse oximeter regularly is important if Covid is suspected. Conditions such as sickle-cell trait should be considered and anybody with such a condition more carefully monitored.

Vaccines

The vaccines are now being administered in the millions and this subject is covered in the next chapter.

Treatment of Post-Covid Exposure

Near the end of July 2021 a cocktail of two monoclonal antibodies was given authorisation by the FDA of the USA for use in people exposed to COVID-19. The two antibodies are casirivimab and imdevimab from Regeneron and this cocktail can be used for treatment or for post-exposure prophylaxis [32]

Conclusion

The pessimism propagated about treatment of COVID-19 was understandable but misguided. Repurposed drugs including oxygen, anti-virals, corticosteroids and other anti-inflammatory agents and anti-coagulants have a major role in treatment of the infection and the inflammatory response. Vitamin D3 is useful in prevention of severe COVID-19 infection.

References

1. https://www.bmj.com/content/369/bmj.m1432 Ferner and Aronson BMJ 2020;369:m1432
2. Rapid Response: Re: Chloroquine and hydroxychloroquine in COVID-19. Goddard, Jarad, Dalgleish https://www.bmj.com/content/369/bmj.m1432/rr-20
3. https://www.recoverytrial.net/results/hydroxychloroquine-results
4. https://www.nursinginpractice.com/clinical/hydroxychloroquine-may-still-be-useful-in-primary-care-covid-treatment-says-lead-scientist/
5. https://www.thelancet.com/pdfs/journals/lanrhe/PIIS2665-9913(20)30378-7.pdf
6. https://www.nihr.ac.uk/news/principle-trial-finds-no-benefit-from-antibiotics-azithromycin-and-doxycycline-for-COVID-19-patients/26680
7. https://www.recoverytrial.net/news/recovery-trial-finds-no-benefit-from-azithromycin-in-patients-hospitalised-with-COVID-19
8. Remdesivir and baricitinib (NEJM) https://www.nejm.org/doi/full/10.1056/NEJMoa2031994
9. https://www.sciencedirect.com/science/article/pii/S2213007120302574
10. Japan https://www.ncbi.nlm.nih.gov/pmc/articles/PMC7467067/
11. India.https://www.pharmaceutical-technology.com/news/glenmark-favipiravir-covid-nod/
12. Russia https://www.contagionlive.com/view/fda-clears-favipiravir-covid19-facility-outbreak-prevention-study
13. acyclovir https://www.researchsquare.com/article/rs-94864/v1
14. https://www.recoverytrial.net/results/dexamethasone-results
15. Hydrocortisone https://www.bmj.com/content/370/bmj.m3472
16. Davidson S and Macleod J, The Principles and Practice of Medicine 10th edition, Churchill and Livingstone 1972 page 429. High dose corticosteroids in circulatory collapse due to severe pneumonia
17. https://www.mirror.co.uk/science/what-dexamethasone-everything-you-need-22200997
18. https://www.recoverytrial.net/news/tocilizumab-reduces-deaths-in-patients-hospitalised-with-COVID-19
19. Davidson S and Macleod J, The Principles and Practice of Medicine 10th edition, Churchill and Livingstone 1972 page 403.
20. https://www.gov.scot/publications/coronavirus-COVID-19-guidance-on-critical-care-management-of-adult-patients/pages/clinical-management-of-pa-

tients-with-COVID-19-infection/
21. Girardis M, Busani S, Damiani E, Donati A, Rinaldi L, Marudi A, et al. Effect of Conservative vs Conventional Oxygen Therapy on Mortality Among Patients in an Intensive Care Unit: The Oxygen-ICU Randomized Clinical Trial. JAMA. 2016 Oct 18;316(15):1583–9
22. Ivermectin trial result: https://www.thelancet.com/journals/eclinm/article/PIIS2589-5370(20)30464-8/fulltext?fbclid=IwAR39IbQQHoadC-7JqP6d8n-kwlVNTQeqaEhrV2qPFJm5ZcjkIKjPD9iQIzx4
23. Amantadine.https://www.pharmacytimes.com/news/evaluating-amantadine-as-a-potential-treatment-for-COVID-19
24. https://www.annalsofoncology.org/article/S0923-7534(20)42464-0/fulltext
25. https://ufhealth.org/news/2020/existing-antihistamine-drugs-show-effectiveness-against-COVID-19-virus-cell-testing
26. https://www.statnews.com/2020/10/01/why-people-with-diabetes-are-being-hit-so-hard-by-COVID-19/
27. https://b-s-h.org.uk/about-us/news/new-data-on-anticoagulants-and-COVID-19/
28. https://www.mainstreetdailynews.com/health/existing-antihistamine-drugs-show-effectiveness-against-COVID-19-virus-in-cell-testing/article_ad7e5610-3672-11eb-b196-a77048777c66.html
29. https://hospitalhealthcare.com/COVID-19/calcifediol-vitamin-d-appears-to-improve-outcomes-in-COVID-19/
30. Vitamin D Deficiency and COVID-19, Anderson and Grimes ISBN 978-0-9562132-7-3
31. https://www.sciencedirect.com/science/article/pii/S2319417020300810oral hygiene and COVID-19
32. www.medpagetoday.com/infectiousdisease/covid19/93844

Acknowledgement: This chapter was prepared in association with Dr Nabil Jarad and Professor Angus Dalgleish

Chapter 16
Vaccines against COVID-19

In December 2019 Peter Daszak was interviewed and stated that it was easy to add spike proteins to harmless coronaviruses and implied that they were infective in humanised mice and therefore also infective in human beings. He also remarked that the team doing this work in Wuhan had also tried to find drugs that would combat the engineered viruses but had no success and that they had tried to make vaccines against the viruses and that this was also a failure.

When the pandemic was announced by the WHO in January 2020 teams of biochemists, pharmacologists and virologists around the world started in earnest to design and make vaccines.

Sorensen and Dalgleish proposed that the perfect vaccine against a coronavirus would aim for the parts that were not human-like and thus would cause the least harmful reaction in human beings [1]. Their vaccine was not chosen for development and investment by the UK Government. Instead they chose the Oxford/AstraZeneca, the Pfizer, the Moderna and the Johnson and Johnson (Janssen) vaccines.

What is the difference between the various vaccines?

Oxford/AstraZeneca, the Pfizer, the Moderna and the Johnson and Johnson (Janssen, J and J) vaccines all contain nucleic acid that codes for the spike proteins of the COVID-19 virus. The differences are mainly in the vector used to get the RNA into the human cells.

The aim has been to get the RNA into muscle cells where it will instruct the cells to make the spike proteins. This is different from a conventional vaccine as the aim is for the person's own cells to make the antigen which will then set off the body's immune response producing a generalised reaction, antibody formation and T cell memory formation.

The usual conventional vaccine consists of the antigen as an attenuated live virus or as a killed virus. This in turn would set off the immune response.

The Pfizer and Moderna vaccines use a lipid shell to surround the mRNA. Oxford/AstraZeneca, Sputnik V (the Russian vaccine) and Johnson and Johnson each use a weakened "harmless" virus as the vector with the genetic code of the harmless adenovirus engineered to produce spike proteins.

The Chinese vaccines Sinovac and Sinopharm use inactivated COVID-19 virus.

By November 2020 trials were well underway and the Pfizer was the first to receive approval for use in the UK. After the results were out I sent an email to Pfizer asking for clarification. I received an automatic reply but nil else.

Pfizer

Email
22/11/2020
To Pfizer Media Relations

Dear Sir/Madam

Re Vaccine against COVID-19

The good news of protection given by your vaccine against COVID-19 has excited people all over the world. But there are also detractors who are totally against vaccination.

I am a retired doctor, medical author of over thirty books and I recently wrote a book about the history of plagues, entitled PANDEMIC. Not surprisingly I am in demand as a speaker on the subject and being asked to write many articles. As someone who is much in favour of vaccines I would like to present your new vaccine in the best possible light.

I have some very specific questions that you may be able to help me with:

The participants
    1.   How many people were enlisted into the trial?
    2.   What were there ages, sex and ethnicity?
    3.   What percentage received a placebo and how comparable were they to those receiving the actual vaccine?
    4.   How many of the people who received the vaccine were asked to return for a second injection and what percentage did return?
    5.   Were the placebo cases invited to return for a second injection and and if so what percentage did return?

Response
    1.   How was response measured?
    2.   What percentages of each of the groups have tested positive for COVID-19?

Adverse reactions
    1.   What adverse reactions were noted? Did the second injection cause more adverse reactions than the first? Were any auto-immune problems encountered?
    2.   Have any of the recipients caught a coronavirus other than COVID-19 and if so what was the severity of the illness.

Background to the science of the vaccine
    1.   I believe that the vaccine is in fact a fragment of mRNA that stimulates the recipient to make the spike proteins which then act as the antigen to which the recipient then responds.

Is this correct and how long does it take for the body to remove the mRNA?

2. What were the results of these novel vaccines in animal experiments?

Storage and administration

1. The storage at very low temperature is critical but at what temperature is the vaccine when administered?

And finally a rather cheeky question that you do not have to answer. Albert Bourla sold 132,508 shares at $41.94 each, according to filings with the US Securities and Exchange Commission, netting a total of around $5.6 million. I have read this was set up in August to occur automatically but that the vaccine was in the offing was known then. What is the view of the Public Relations department on this embarrassing occurrence? Does it imply that Bouria believes the increase in share price will not last?

Answers to these questions would be very much welcomed and may set the minds of many people at ease.

Kind regards
Professor Paul R Goddard MD, FRCR, FBIR

23/11/2020
To Pfizer Media Relations
Dear Sir/Madam
I have added one more question
Worst-case scenario

In the latest New Scientist (21 Nov 2020) the possibility is raised that a vaccine could reduce disease such that it became sub-clinical but still permit viral shedding. Has this possibility been considered and how frequent was Covid testing of asymptomatic volunteers?

Kind regards Paul Goddard

Automatic reply
22/11/2020

Hello, Thank you for contacting Pfizer Media Relations. Your inquiry was received and we will be responding as soon as possible. If you are a journalist with an urgent inquiry, please call the Pfizer Media Relations line at 212-733-1226. If you are not a working member of the media, we will do our best to forward your inquiry to the appropriate contact at Pfizer, but you will not receive a reply from us.

Best regards, Pfizer Media Relations

23/7/2021
Dear Pfizer Media Relations
Hi
I have still received no reply to my questions sent in November last year and would appreciate a suitable response. Yours faithfully   Paul R Goddard

The questions remain relevant and are still unanswered by the company.

It appears that they know next to nothing about the pharmacokinetics of the various vaccines but they have received approval on the basis of the overlapping phased trials and approval for vaccines rather than for gene therapy.

What is said to be in the vaccines
and what is rumoured to be in them?

There is a lot of conjecture about the various vaccines and what is reckoned to be in them. Some people claim to have noticed that a fridge magnet would stick to the site of their vaccination. No such luck in my own case : I tried it but the magnet did not stick to my arm.

One theory being put around is that the vaccine shot includes a microchip. This is entirely implausible because of the very small size of the injected volume.

"Each dose of the University of Oxford/AstraZeneca vaccine is 0.5 milliliters, and each dose of the Pfizer/BioNTech vaccine is 0.3 millitres. The active ingredients in these vaccines amount to just a few thousandths of a gram."

Having received no reply from Pfizer I have gleaned this information from the internet.[1]

Pfizer vaccine content:
mRNA molecules enclosed in tiny fatty spheres
ALC-0315 = (4-hydroxybutyl)azanediyl)bis(hexane-6,1-diyl) bis(2-hexyldecanoate)
ALC-0159 = 2[(polyethylene glycol)-2000]-N,N-ditetradecylacetamide
1,2-Distearoyl-sn-glycero-3-phosphocholine
cholesterol
Salts:
- potassium chloride
- potassium dihydrogen phosphate
- sodium chloride
- disodium hydrogen phosphate dihydrate

Sugar: sucrose

Other theories are that it contains iron. Nanoparticles of iron have previously been proposed as an adjunct for vaccines but are not included on the product data sheets and are unlikely to be present.

Another suggestion is that the vaccine contains graphene. That is harder to dismiss as the fatty shells could include a precursor for graphene. The little lipid balls which contain the mRNA are only about the size of a virus.

I have suggested that the magnet test should be carried out on the arm immediately after injection. If the susceptibility is due to an injected compound of iron or graphene the injection site theoretically should cause immediate attraction. If the attraction develops over a few hours then it is probably due to haematoma development due to bleeding from a small blood vessel. Of course it is entirely possible that the magnet videos are simply a hoax but I have no evidence either way.

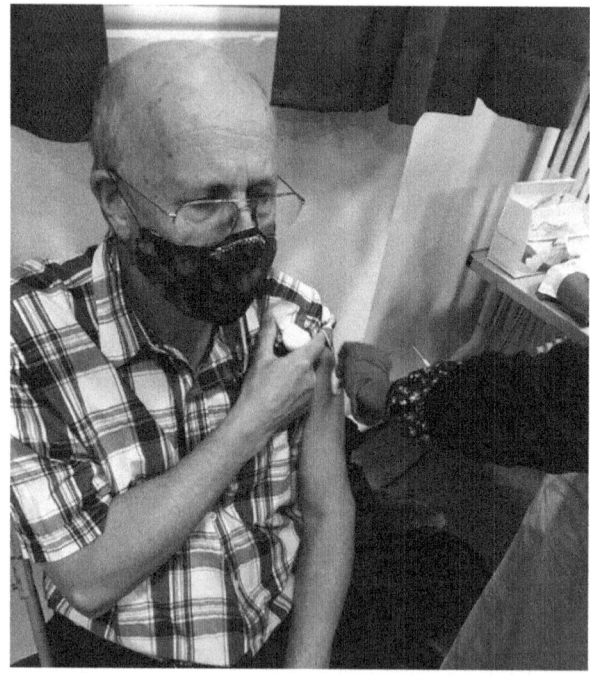

Taking the Jab. (Astra/Zeneca)

My body language tells me that I was feeling rather apprehensive.

I did feel very grateful to the volunteers who were manning the place.

Astra/Zeneca

Here I am taking my first jab of the AstraZeneca vaccine. This vaccine costs about £1 compared with the Pfizer at £20 per shot. The AZ vaccine uses technology known as the ChAdOx1 which was developed by the Jenner Institute which is based within the Nuffield Department of Medicine, Oxford University.

The results from the interim trials in 23,000 people in the UK, Brazil and South Africa showed that the AstraZeneca vaccine protected over 70% of recipients. Results from the roll out of the vaccine show that it gives a greater than 90% protection against the need for hospitalisation with Covid.

Even with the latest variants in the UK the prevalence of the viral infection is three times greater in the unvaccinated than the vaccinated.

The Pfizer vaccine is said to have had even greater effect in preventing hospitalisation due to infection.

The roll out of the vaccines started in the UK in late December 2020 just as the third wave was underway. The third wave peaked in January 2021 and was then pushed down by the dramatic and successful vaccine programme

Vaccine Side Effects

Side effects due to vaccines are not at all uncommon whatever disease is being vaccinated against and whichever vaccine is used.

In the case of the COVID-19 vaccines the first serious side-effect noted has been blood clots due to the AstraZeneca vaccine. These have been venous in nature with 11 excess events per 100,000 cases [2] and around twice as many venous clots as would be expected in the normal population. The greatest danger was from cerebral venous thrombosis and overall about 1 in 250,000 died as a result. The danger from getting COVID-19 is much greater than the danger from the AZ vaccine for people over 50 years old but in younger people the risk/benefit ratio is not so favourable so the use of the AstraZeneca vaccine in young people has been suspended in favour of the Pfizer vaccine. Public Health England have stated that similar problems have occurred with the Johnson and Johnson (Janssen) vaccine which also uses an adenovirus vector. The problem is worsened by heparin but may be improved by the use of non-heparin anti-coagulants including low dose gastro-resistant aspirin (usually 75mg per day). D Dimer studies which demonstrate the presence of thrombosis have also been positive in a high proportion of recipients of other vaccines and fibrinogen may be low.

Common side-effects due to the vaccines have been reported anecdotally to include a sore arm at the site of injection, muscle aches, tiredness, headache, feeling or being sick. Slight fever and a shivery feeling for 1 or 2 days are also fairly common. These effects occur in as many as 10% or more and the headaches occur in half the recipients.

Uncommonly the vaccine may cause a severe anaphylactic reaction and any history of a reaction from the first injection mitigates against repeated vaccination.

The long term effects are, as yet, unknown as the pharmacology is so new.

New Variants

I have discussed the advent of new variants in a previous chapter. AstraZeneca and Pfizer in the UK have been shown to be effective in reducing the need for hospitalisation due to COVID-19. The South African variant (Beta) is more resistant to the vaccine response but has mostly been chased away in the UK by the Delta variant (Indian).

The Chinese Sinovac vaccine was distributed very successfully in Chile. Unfortunately it has not proven to give protection against new variants including, recently, the Lamda variant that was first identified in Peru. Now Chile have gone from being the poster boy of vaccination programmes to a disaster zone, from hero to zero.

Booster Vaccines

The WHO recently called for a moratorium on booster jabs in countries such as the UK where most of the older adults have already had their first two vaccine doses. They want the rest of the world to catch up and do not want all the vaccines taken up by the rich countries.

I, for entirely different reasons, feel that booster jabs are not yet appropriate. As discussed by Sorensen and Dalgleish in their seminal paper [4], the spike protein vaccines have inherent dangers and limited usefulness because the spike proteins are constantly changing. They suggest that the parts of the virus that are preserved are the bits that the vaccine should be aiming at and constantly boosting the immune system against self-like spike proteins does risk an increasing number of auto-immune reactions. The presently available vaccines certainly reduce the severity of the illness but the fully vaccinated can still catch variants of the disease. Using the present vaccines it is highly unlikely that we will ever reach herd immunity even if nearly everybody is vaccinated.[5]

References
1. https://practio.co.uk/coronavirus/articles/coronavirus-vaccine-ingredients
2. BMJ report 6/5/2021
3. Blood Clotting following COVID-19 Vaccination: Public Health England 2021
4. Sørensen B, Susrud A, Dalgleish AG (2020). Biovacc-19: A Candidate Vaccine for COVID-19 (SARS-CoV-2) Developed from Analysis of its General Method of Action for Infectivity. QRB Discovery, 1: e6, 1–11 https://doi.org/10.1017/qrd.2020.8
5. Herd immunity to covid-19 may not be attainable in the UK. Helen Thomson, New Scientist, 21 August 2021, p17

Chapter 17
Antibiotics and Vaccination lead to Complacency
The Discovery of Penicillin

Once upon a time in 1928 an astonishingly lucky chance discovery by Alexander Fleming led to the amazing medical nirvana of the antibiotic era. And we all lived happily ever after.

Or did he and did we? Well, that's the fairy tale that Fleming and St Mary's would like us to believe, similar in its nature to the apple falling on the receptive head of Newton or the overflowing bath of Archimedes and his accompanying cry of "Eureka!"

Sir Alexander Fleming is lauded by many as the great discoverer of antibiotics. Apparently a petri dish containing a staphylococcal culture was left on a lab bench and a penicillium mould spore floated onto the dish. Fleming was away for two weeks and on his return he observed that the growth of the staphylococcus had been inhibited by the penicillium. He photographed the petri dish and told the world of his discovery.

But was this really true and did people already know that some moulds inhibited bacterial growth?

The story told by Fleming was contradictory and he had, for years, been working systematically through various moulds and bacterial growths. The laboratory on the floor below was working on moulds and as far back as the 19th century antagonism between bacteria and moulds had been observed and called "antibiosis". British physiologist John Scott Burdon-Sanderson in 1870, almost 60 years before Fleming's finding, had published a paper on the phenomenon. Folk

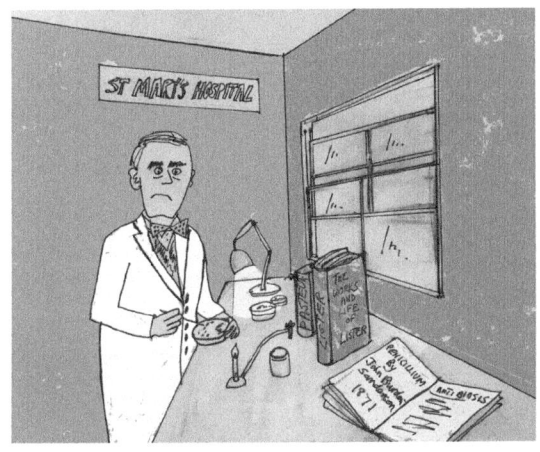

Alexander Fleming at work in his laboratory in St Mary's Hospital. The works of John Scott Burdon-Sanderson, Lister and Pasteur are all available on his desk.

(Photographs don't show these works but Fleming must have been aware of them so I've taken the liberty of adding them).

Note the open window through which the spores are apocryphally supposed to have travelled.

tradition used moulds in medicine and grooms were well known to use mouldy bread for treating wounds on horses' legs and both Pasteur and Lister researched into antibiosis.[1,2] I reckon that he felt obliged to keep to the serendipity story and that was the reason that he always looked so cross. The "sheer luck" aspect denigrated a lot of the hard work he had been doing.

So it is more likely that Fleming was purposely working on the moulds and staphylococcus knowing that antibiosis occurred. His paper on the subject was published in the British Journal of Experimental Pathology in June 1929 and more or less ignored until Howard Walter Florey and Ernst Boris Chain ten years later managed to isolate and purify the substance that Fleming had called "penicillin".

They went on to produce sufficient quantities to initially test it in mice and then in two human beings. The first was an unfortunate woman who was dying from cancer and volunteered to test the new drug. She had a bad reaction to impurities in the preparation. The second patient, a policeman with a serious facial infection from a cut suffered during a German bombing raid, was more lucky initially and showed a good response but the team ran out of the penicillin preparation and the patient relapsed and died.[3]

Florey and Chain could not produce enough of the penicillin so they went over to the USA where the stuff was produced in industrial quantities by a fermentation process. They finally had sufficient to use in patients and they started to trial it in the battlefield hospitals of the second world war. Florey flew back to England to lead the clinical trials that eventually took him as far afield as North Africa and to our then ally, the Soviet Union.[3]

SECTION 28.

SOFT TISSUE WOUNDS AT NO. 71 GENERAL HOSPITAL.

Captain G. K. Tutton.

Case	Site	Size	Age	Penicillin	Healing
1. Lt.-Cdr. A.	Abd. wall	5 × 3 cm.	4 hrs.	Solution	Complete union
	Forearm	6 cm.	4 hrs.	> 27,500 U.	Complete union
	Forearm	6 cm.	4 hrs.	3 days'	Complete union
	Chest wall	12 cm.	4 hrs.	Powder	Complete union
	Amput. finger		4 hrs.	Powder	Incomplete union
2. Pte. J.	Thigh	5 × 2 cm.	7 hrs.	Solution 84,500 U.	Complete union
	Thigh	7 × 3 cm.	7 hrs.	4 days	Complete union (Subsequent small abscess in wound due to *B. pyocyaneus*.)
3. Pte. D.	Shoulder	9 × 6 cm.	3½ days	Solution 7,250 U. 3 days	Complete union
4. Lt. E.	Forearm		4 days	Powder	Complete union
	Upper arm		4 days	Powder	Incomplete union
5. Pte. D.	Back	6 × 3 cm.	5 days	Powder	Complete union
	Back	?	5 days	Powder	Incomplete union
6. Pte. R.	Shoulder	6 cm.	5 days	Powder	Complete union
7. P.O.W.	Amput. upper thigh			Solution (local) 47,500 U.	Wound at first left open. Prompt healing after secondary suture
	Septicaemia		10 days	Na. Pen. I.M. & I.V. 270,000 U.	Recovery from septicaemia.

Case 2 in the above table is of particular interest as the first case from the Battle of Sicily in which wounds were closed with the aid of penicillin.

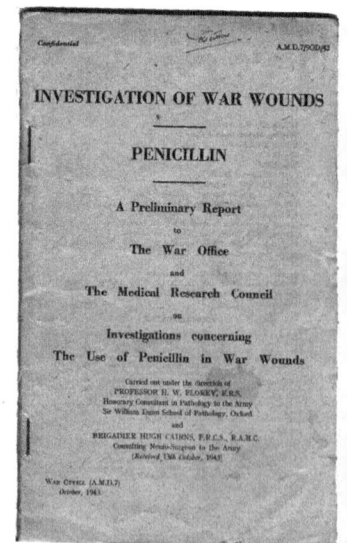

Confidential A.M.D.7/9OD/43

INVESTIGATION OF WAR WOUNDS

PENICILLIN

A Preliminary Report

to

The War Office
and
The Medical Research Council

on

Investigations concerning
The Use of Penicillin in War Wounds

Carried out under the direction of
PROFESSOR H. W. FLOREY, F.R.S.
Honorary Consultant in Pathology to the Army
Sir William Dunn School of Pathology, Oxford

and

BRIGADIER HUGH CAIRNS, F.R.C.S., R.A.M.C.
Consulting Neuro-Surgeon to the Army
(Retired 15th October, 1943)

War Office (A.M.D.7)
October, 1943

My father-in-law, Ken Tutton, was a surgeon in the RAMC at the time and participated in the trials of penicillin in North Africa. Lois Tutton states 'My father's contribution to this report was a section on "Soft tissue Wounds at 71 General Hospital."' [4,5]

The report set the protocol for the use of penicillin for the rest of the war.

The structure of penicillin was analysed by Dorothy Hodgkin but chemical synthesis of penicillin was not achieved until 1957 and the fermentation method of production was maintained well beyond that date.

Substances that could fight infectious diseases in vivo were known before the advent of penicillin. In the section on syphilis I mentioned mercury and arsenicals, both very toxic. In the 1930s the sulphonamides were discovered in Germany but Penicillin was better than all of these.

The era of antibiotics to fight infections had begun and very soon people began to be blasé about infections and started feeding antibiotics to cattle as growth promoters.

Immunisations could be used against most viral diseases and bacterial infections could be treated with antibiotics so what was there to fear?

The elimination of smallpox from the world, announced in 1979, added to this pride in the achievements of medical science. At least in the developed world we felt safe from the ravages of infection.

The AIDS Epidemic

This complacency was shattered in the early 1980s with the AIDS epidemic which was discussed in chapter 9. However the lack of early testing, quarantining and contact tracing for COVID-19 coronavirus in this recent pandemic shows that we have not learnt the lessons of history. I mentioned to another doctor very early on in the pandemic that patients and contacts should have been quarantined in isolation hospitals. He replied that he did not think that the public nowadays would have put up with that. Instead we have all been quarantined half-heartedly and the economy has, at least for the time being, been decimated.

Antibiotic Resistant Bugs

Feeding antibiotics to cattle as growth promoters and the availability of antibiotics over the counter in many countries has inevitably led to widespread antibiotic-resistance so this has added to the rebirth of fear of infection.

Methicillin resistant *Staph. aureus* (MRSA) infection and *Clostridium difficile* are two hospital-acquired infections that reached almost epidemic proportions some fifteen or twenty years ago. Now people realise that hospitals are not the safe havens they used to consider them to be.

The development of new antibiotics has been hampered by the way in which the drug companies making novel medicines are remunerated. This is almost exclusively by the capitalist system of profit-making which is thought to be the most effective way of stimulating research and development in the developed world. It is not, however, the only way as the development of Artemesinin showed (see chapter 3).

The problem is this. When a new medicine is developed it takes years of research and major clinical trials, and costs billions of dollars. Then there is only a short time during which the drug is under patent and the drug company must recoup their outgoing costs and make a profit. New antibiotics are usually kept in reserve by the doctors until they find that the presently tried and tested antibiotics are not working or that the bug is resistant to them. Then they might use one of the new antibiotics. In most cases this will not be the case and by the time the bugs are generally resistant to the old drugs the new antibiotic is out of patent and any company can make it. Hence the originating pharmaceutical company will not make a profit. Add to that the fact that when they do develop a new anti-malarial or anti-whatever and it is found to be essential there is an outcry if they don't give it away to the Third World that is crying out for it for nothing.

The present system works well for research into diseases of the rich. In fact the world's dominant superpower, the USA, produces wonderful medical research into diseases of the rich. Unfortunately the majority of the world, and even the majority of people in the United States, are poor and this is particularly the case when it comes to the huge private bills that even a short stay in an American hospital cost.

At present the hospitals are working at a very low capacity due to the COVID-19 corona virus pandemic. Various drugs are being trialled but the public are fervently hoping for a vaccine. Once again I worry that a vaccine may cause similar problems to the AIDS vaccines. So that brings us to the next subject.

Vaccination

Edward Jenner's starring role in the development of vaccination has been stressed in an earlier chapter. Certainly the eradication of smallpox has saved many millions of lives and possibly billions of people from hideously deforming scars. It was by far the most successful intervention of medical science. Ever!

Jenner's success led to a search for vaccines against many common infectious diseases. Pasteur was next when he discovered a vaccine against anthrax and an attenuated live vaccine against rabies.

Vaccines against twenty-six different infections (and multiple versions of each) are available and used in the USA ranging from Adenovirus to Yellow Fever. Many othe vaccines exist but are not on the commonly used list. I, for example, had a vaccine against bubonic plague (see chapter 4).

But vaccination and all types of immunisation have a very chequered history.

The proponents of vaccination against smallpox claimed throughout the 19th century that it was harmless, safe and gave lifelong immunity against smallpox. In fact there are many people who needed to avoid vaccination (for example, people with eczema) and the immunity probably lasts ten years, not a lifetime, then a booster is required to maintain the immunity.

Syphilisation in the 19th century was an example of extremely poor medical practice with doctors carrying out prolonged and repeated inoculation of supposedly attenuated syphilitic matter into patients who already were suffering from the disease. By all accounts it only served to make matters worse.

There are occasions in which the vaccines have been contaminated or harmful in other ways and the longterm effects of modern vaccines are only now being determined.

Overall for the human race vaccines have been an amazing boon but for an individual they have sometimes been disastrous.

The Wakefield Affair

It is very difficult to write about this without upsetting one side or other on this debate. Putting people off having their children vaccinated risks major epidemics that can otherwise be avoided but, and it is a big but, vaccination does carry some risk whatever the vaccinationists may say to the contrary.

So what happened? In 1998 Andrew Wakefield presented a paper in the Lancet that purported to show the MMR vaccine (measles, mumps and rubella) causing a new sydrome of autism and bowel disease. This was later retracted and Wakefield was struck off the British Medical Register.

Was there any truth in the assertion?

Research has now shown that there is a reduced chance of autism in vaccinated children compared with children who are not vaccinated which appears to suggest that the Lancet paper was completely incorrect.

The argument is rather more nuanced than this. Yes, overall it is safer to be vaccinated but an individual could still suffer from having an immunisation and it is the individual cases that make the news.

Combined MMR vaccines have been in trouble from the very beginning.

In September 1992 the Department of Health withdrew two brands of MMR vaccine after research suggested they were associated with a raised incidence of transient mumps meningitis, although much lower than with natural disease.[10]

Wakefield has never suggested that vaccination should stop...he has always called for the introduction of separate vaccines for each of measles, mumps and rubella. Whether they would be safer than the joint vaccine is not known.

In 2004 it was revealed that the Legal Aid Board funded Wakefield's research and that many of the children in the report were litigants. This was clearly a vested interest and in March of 2004 ten of the thirteen authors withdrew their support for Wakefield's paper.

A measles outbreak occurred in the UK in 2006 and one child died, the first for 14 years. In 2010 the paper was withdrawn by the Lancet and Wakefield was struck off.

But is it possible that vaccinations could cause the syndrome Wakefield described? Well, yes. Even the makers of the vaccines never say they are completely safe....just that they are safer than catching the disease. That much is definitely true and it is possible that they could be made even safer but once again, as with antibiotics, we come across cost/benefit analysis and lack of profit as a reason for not creating new versions of the vaccines.

"Public confidence in MMR and vaccination has never fully recovered, at least not in developed countries. This was made evident by recent news that the number of measles cases in Europe increased by 400 per cent in 2017, with more than 20,000 cases and 35 needless deaths." [10]

Reports published by the Centers for Disease Control (CDC) and the National Center for Biotechnology Information (NCBI) state that the following vaccines have been linked to encephalitis:[11]

- MMR vaccine – Measles, Mumps and Rubella
- DTP or DTaP vaccine – Diphtheria, Tetanus, and Pertussis (whooping cough).
- Influenza (flu) vaccine

Some of these vaccines have also been associated with conditions similar to secondary encephalitis, such as acute disseminated encephalomyelitis (ADEM) and measles inclusion body encephalitis.

There have been more than 1,100 cases of encephalitis (including brain stem encephalitis) reported to the Vaccine Adverse Event Reporting System (VAERS).[11]

If everybody in the USA is being vaccinated that makes encephalitis an event that occurs in about 1 in 300,000 people. Many are vaccinated multiple times bringing this down to the ballpark figure of one in a million.

Note that the chance of dying from a measles epidemic is somewhere between one in six hundred and one in a thousand. Clearly it is safer to be vaccinated than to suffer from an epidemic.

But we have always known that it is better to be vaccinated and before there were vaccination programs careful parents tried to make sure that their children had the childhood illnesses when they were fit, healthy children.

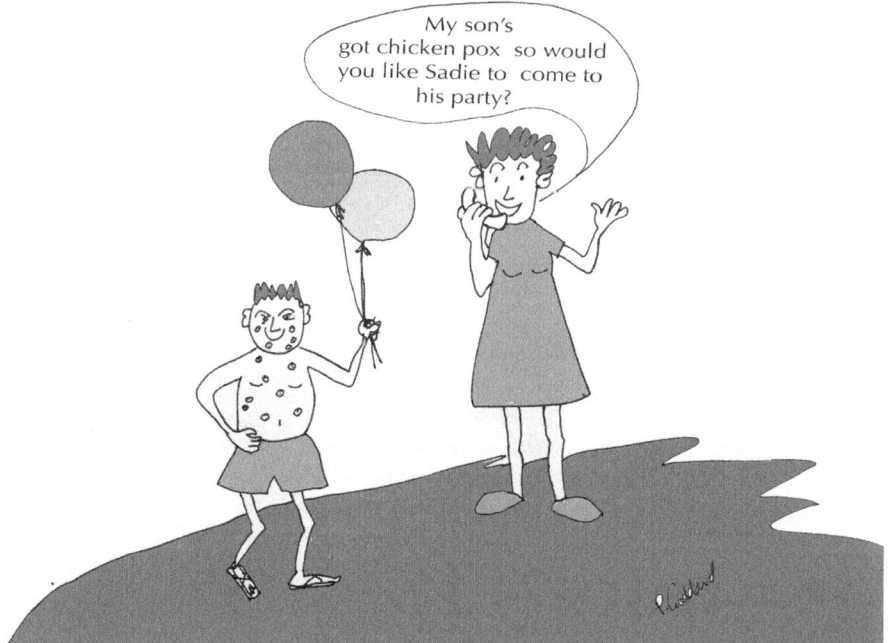

So what is the advice to parents? If your child is ill, wait until he or she is better before having a vaccination. Who else should not be vaccinated? That depends on the vaccine concerned and the guidelines are too long and detailed to be included here. They can be found online. [12] The type of advice is to avoid vaccination if they are the wrong age or if there was a previous allergic reaction, recent coma, seizures etc.

Some people will not want their children to be vaccinated at all. They are then relying on the herd immunity provided by other people's children being vaccinated and this could result in some hostility if the parents of the other children get to hear about the decision, though they are probably not putting vaccinated children at greater risk. Moreover it is possible that lack of vaccination could debar a person from travelling abroad or working in certain health care occupations. With regard to COVID-19 the appearance of multiple variants which vaccinated people can catch means that total herd immunity is unlikely to be achieved by vaccination. The subject of vaccination for COVID-19 was also discussed in chapter 16.

References

1. https://www.sciencehistory.org/historical-profile/alexander-fleming
2. https://www.bbvaopenmind.com/en/science/bioscience/fleming-and-the-difficult-beginnings-of-penicillin-myth-and-reality/
3. https://www.sciencehistory.org/historical-profile/howard-walter-florey-and-ernst-boris-chain
4. Lois Tutton, personal communication
5. Neurosurgery and the North Africa Campaign in World War 2 L M Tutton BDS, MSc September 2011 Bristol Medico-Historical Society Proceedings Volume VI
6. https://en.wikipedia.org/wiki/Angus_Dalgleish "produced the first link between Slim Disease and HIV infection."
7. https://www.nhsinform.scot/illnesses-and-conditions/cancer/cancer-types-in-adults/kaposis-sarcoma
8. Key HIV trial in South Africa ends because of poor results, The Guardian 3.2.2020
9. https://www.thelancet.com/journals/lancet/article/PIIS0140-6736(00)04536-0/fulltext#article_upsell
10. https://www.independent.co.uk/life-style/health-and-families/health-news/timeline-how-the-andrew-wakefield-mmr-vaccine-scare-story-spread-8570591.html
11. https://www.mctlaw.com/vaccine-injury/encephalitis-vaccine-reaction/
12. https://www.cdc.gov/vaccines/vpd/should-not-vacc.html

Chapter 18
A Far Future Plague?

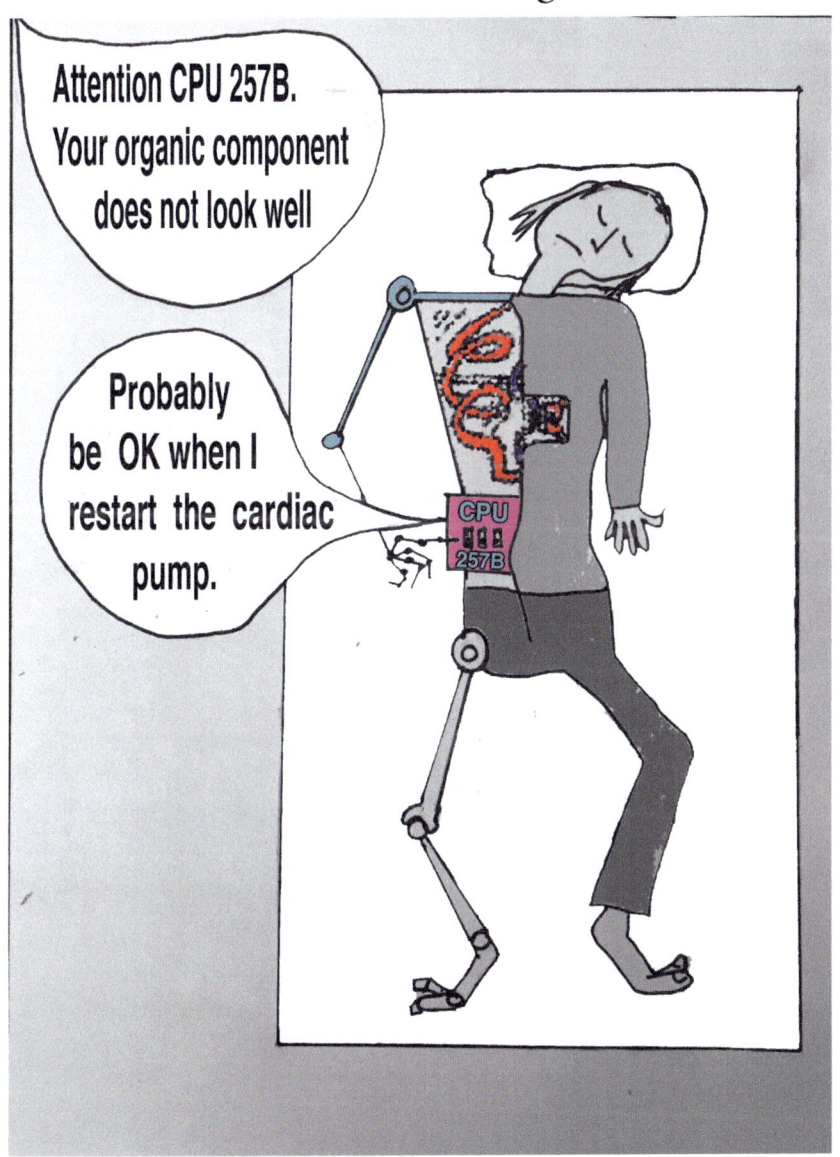

A computer virus has infected the central processing unit of the cyborg and made it rather indifferent to the fate of the organic components.

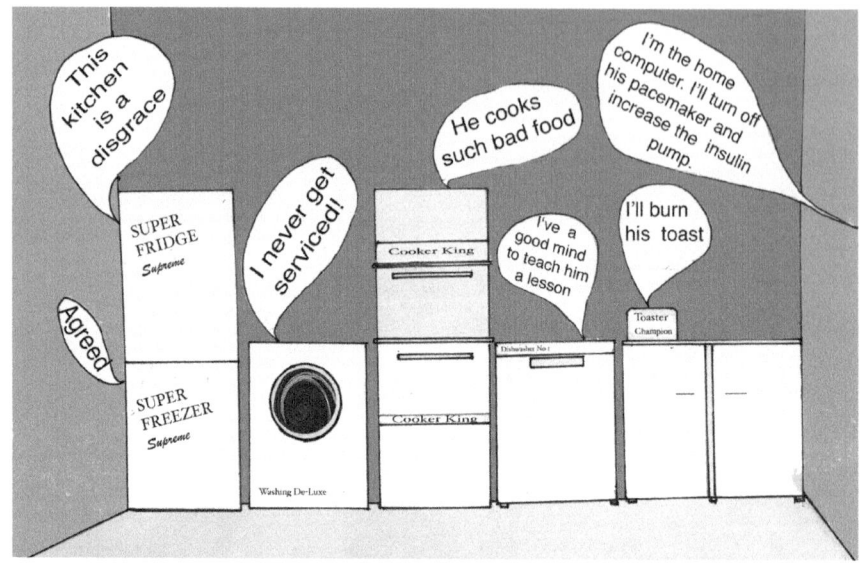

Malware in the Kitchen

The threat of a software virus plague hitting our cyborg selves may seem a science fiction fantasy but it is closer to reality than we like to think. Consider what would happen if a hacker, malware or a virus got into the "Internet of Things" in your kitchen.

OK, the home computer, the pacemaker and insulin pump are not necessarily in the kitchen. But can they be hacked or infected with a virus? What is the chance that our 'white ware' will turn against us?

The answer is twofold. Yes, our 'internet of things' is absurdly easy to hack into and, yes, already it has already been turned against us. At the moment I only have evidence of hackers purposely affecting our health care rather than the computer system itself doing the dirty on us. But what an example!

In May 2017 I was preparing the Long Fox lecture for November that year and I had produced some slides about far future pandemics and plagues. I considered that computer viruses would become more important in health care in the future. Little did I realise that within a few days the prediction would come true. It was reported at the time that forty-eight British health care systems were attacked by a hacker's virus. 130,000 IT systems across the globe were affected. Ninety-nine countries were simultaneously asked for ransom money by the hacker and tens of thousands of pounds had already been paid.

Routine NHS work had to be cancelled until the MRI machines, CT scanners and other vital equipment were repaired.

By the end of October it was possible to look back with hindsight and realise

NHS cyber chaos hits thousands of patients

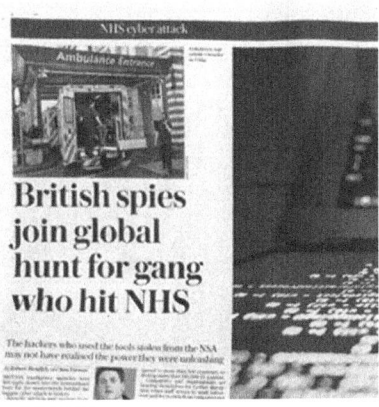

Sunday Telegraph May 14 2017

that the so-called 'WannaCry' hack of the NHS could have been avoided with basic IT security.

The National Audit Office (NAO) reported that 19,500 medical appointments were cancelled, computers at 600 GP surgeries were locked and five hospitals had to divert ambulances elsewhere. [1]

MRI and CT machines although sophisticated pieces of equipment usually incorporate slave computers in their workings and they are inevitably old tech by the time the machine is sold. 37 NHS trusts were eventually affected.

NHS Digital had carried out security checks on the computer systems of more than a third of the NHS trusts in England before the hacking attack and none, not one, had passed. Remedial action had not been taken in most of the trusts.

A Russian hacking group called The Shadow Brokers were suspected of leaking the method of hacking which had been stolen from the NSA but the group actually making the attack were almost certainly from North Korea. It eventually reached 150 countries, three-quarters of the countries in the world! The damage could have been worse if a young security researcher, Marcus Hutchins, had not found a method of stopping the virus by activating a "kill switch."

Once human beings are irrevocably linked to chips a computer virus could kill them. And surprisngly enough many are already linked to computers. In 2009 the 500,000th pacemaker was fitted.[2]

That number has now risen to one million a year. In addition 200,000 defibrillators are fitted annually. Insulin pumps, controlled by a chip or two measuring blood sugar, are in use worldwide. York hospital recently reported that they have 280 patients on such pumps. Hundreds of thousands of cochlear implants are in use worldwide.[3]

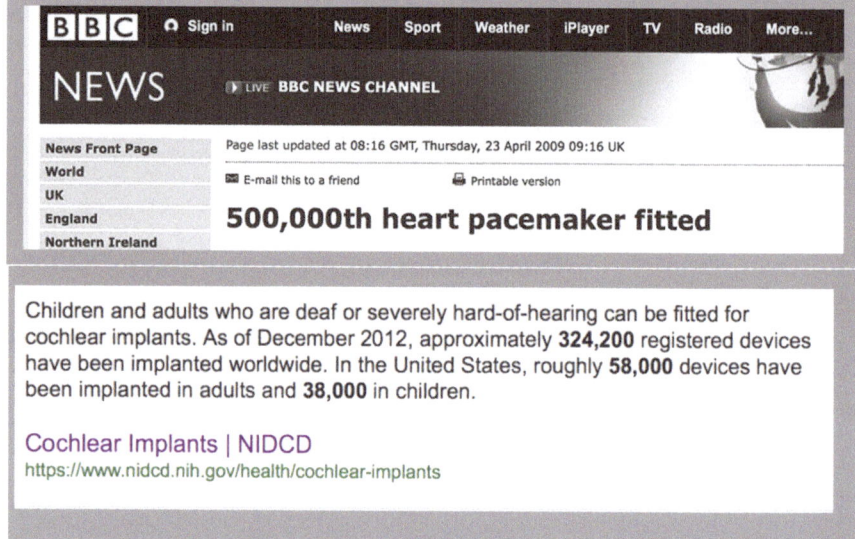

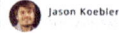

A variety of brain implants have been developed for control of Parkinson's Disease and epilepsy.

All the implants are said to be easily hacked[4] which probably led to MJ Marazan, the science fiction writer, penning the short story that finished the first edition of this book. In this edition we have, instead, conclusions and suggestions.

References

1. https://www.theguardian.com/technology/2017/oct/27/nhs-could-have-avoided-wannacry-hack-basic-it-security-national-audit-office
2. 500,000 pacemaker fitted, BBC News 23rd April 2009
3. Cochlear implants www.nidcd.nih.gov/health/cochlear-implants
4. https://www.vice.com/en_us/article/kbzmbz/hackers-killed-a-simulated-human-by-turning-off-its-pacemakerdictionary.com>).

Conclusions and Suggestions

We are now almost two years into a worldwide pandemic. Are we very much further forward in dealing with it and what should be done?

Firstly we must face facts.

- The COVID-19 coronavirus was adapted in a laboratory from a precursor bat coronavirus and it escaped. This was due to the hubris of scientists thinking that they could safely adapt the viruses. The history of multiple escapes from laboratories shows that they cannot. The Gain of Function studies which make harmless viruses into pathogens must stop now worldwide.
- The Chinese Communist Party and its leaders, the Americans and others who backed the Wuhan research need to face court action.
- The cover-ups and lies from scientists and politicians must stop and scientific debate must be encouraged. Science has suffered a terrible blow to its credibility due to the escape of the virus, the cover-ups and the predictions that failed to materialise. This has further divided society. There are now people who consider all of the scientific pronouncements as lies and others who think that the development of the vaccines have made the virologists into heroes. We need to thank all the volunteers who helped roll out the vaccination programme in the UK but it is true that the vaccines would not have been needed if the virus had never been developed.
- The medical practitioners must be permitted clinical freedom to use all available and prescribable drugs for their sick patients. The managers and politicians, chief medical officers and executive officers should not be ruling the roost. Guidelines should not be used as directives. In the case of COVID-19 there are many drugs and supplements that can be beneficial and many people believe, perhaps correctly, that they were not being promoted because the big pharmaceutical companies could not make a profit from them. A method of financing the development of new anti-virals, antibiotics and supplements should be deployed that does not rely on making vast profits during a period of exclusive ownership of the patents and copyrights. Charity and government-backed prizes may be a partial answer. Politicians and managers need to be governed by an equivalent body to the General Medical Council (GMC).
- Cybersecurity of the "internet of things" must be made a priority.

Index

AIDS (HIV)	15, 82-84	Mendeleev	57
Alzheimer's disease	87-90	MERS	119
Anthrax	43	NHS Computer hack	166-167
Antibiotics	157	Pandemic; definition	13
Apocalypse	10	Pandemic; worst	14-17
Artemesinin	27	PCP pneumonia	82
Black Death	16, 32	PCR	10
Bubonic plague	10, 16, 30	Penicillin	163-165
Budd, William	42, 73	Plague of Athens	72
Cholera	15, 43, 72	Plague; definition	13
Chopin	43	Pneumocystis carinii	82
Coronaviruses	17, 91-93	Poliomyelitis	
COVID-19	10, 91-162	(infantile paralysis)	17, 58, 59
Diarrhoea and dysentery	71, 79	Porphyromonas gingivalis	87
Diphtheria	17	Pott's disease	
Ebola	11, 17, 86	(spinal tuberculosis)	40-41
Fleming, Alexander	155	Quarantine	10
Florence Nightingale	74, 75	Rabbit hemorrhagic virus	67
Florey and Chain	158	SARS	119
Great fire of London	34	SARS 2 see COVID-19	
Great plague of London	34	Scarlet Fever	10, 17, 68
Guillain-Barré syndrome	59, 60	Scrofula (cervical node TB)	45-48
Heaf test	51	Sepsis	66-68
Hepatitis	14, 85	Simian Immuno Deficiency Virus	
HIV (AIDS)	15	(SIV)	83-84
Hubris, scientific	10	Smallpox	10, 16, 20
Influenza	15, 53	Snow, John	72
Jenner, Edward	22	Syphilis	10, 15, 61
Justinian plague	30	Third Pandemic of plague	37
King's Evil, see Scrofula		Tracing App	35
Leprosy	10, 64-66	Trump, Donald	9, 10,
Long Fox, Edward	9	Tuberculosis	10, 16, 40
Lyme Disease	17, 63	Tuberculosis, military	43
Mad cow disease	87	Typhoid	17, 72-77
Malaria	16, 26	Typhus	15, 77, 78
Man Flu	55-56	Vaccination	167-170
Marburg virus	86	War and plagues	18
Measles	17	Yellow fever	17

There is more about COVID-19 in a new book *"The Origin of the Virus"* by Paolo Barnard, Steven Quay and Angus Dalgleish. (isbn 9781854571069)